'HE WENT ABOUT DOING GOOD'

D Elder

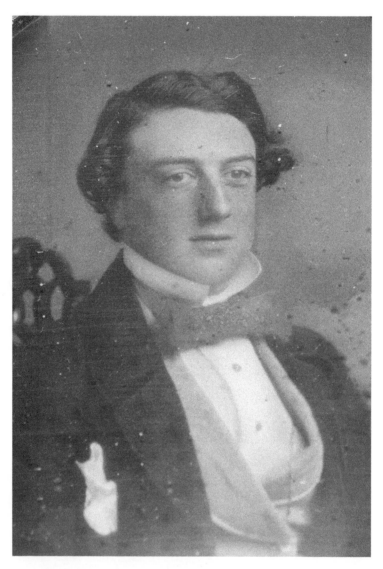

Detail from a hand-coloured daguerreotype of ETW, by Richard Lowe
(Cheltenham Borough Council and the Cheltenham Trust/The
Wilson Family Collection). See p. 36.

'HE WENT ABOUT DOING GOOD'

The Life of
Dr Edward Thomas Wilson
of Cheltenham
(1832-1918)

DAVID ELDER

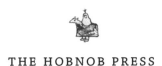

THE HOBNOB PRESS

First published in the United Kingdom
by The Hobnob Press,
8 Lock Warehouse, Severn Road, Gloucester GL1 2GA
www.hobnobpress.co.uk

British Library Cataloguing in Publication Data
A catalogue record for this book is available from the British Library

ISBN 978-1-914407-25-3

Typeset in Chapparal Pro 11/14 pt
Typesetting and origination by John Chandler

Cover illustrations
    Front: ETW with tripod, c.1892.
    Back: Detail from a portrait of ETW by Alfred Soord. See p. 167.
        (both Cheltenham Borough Council and the Cheltenham Trust/The Wilson Family Collection).

    Inside covers: Details from 'The Crippetts'. 1898. Drawing by Ted Wilson
        (Cheltenham College Archives).

Contents

To
Edward Thomas Wilson and his descendants,
who have contributed to the life of Cheltenham
for the past 150 years

Foreword

SOME GREAT ACHIEVERS of public good attain celebrity, wealth or power; others accomplish as much but remain hidden in the shadows, their influence touching our everyday lives but rarely acknowledged. Such a man was my great grandfather, Edward Thomas Wilson, whose effect on the development of modern Cheltenham and the everyday lives of its citizens remains palpable, more than a century after his death. He was the GP for many in the Town, yet also a pioneer of photomicrography, of modern medical practice, of clean drinking water, of the conservation movement, of public libraries and he led the campaign for the foundation of the Town Museum, which he opened in 1907. His work to combat epidemics in the Town, through the promotion of vaccination and isolation fever hospitals seems, in 2021, alarmingly contemporary, as do many of his papers to the Cheltenham Natural Science Society of which he was President for many years.

Yet for all his pioneering achievement, he always felt himself overshadowed by other family members, in particular, his brother, a noted explorer of the Holy Land, who was sent to rescue Gordon at Khartoum; and his son, a noted explorer of the Antarctic, who died with Captain Scott. To them went the public recognition, the honours, the titles, the medals and the memorials; to him went obscurity. This finally changed in 2012, almost a century after his death, when by public acclaim *The Cheltenham Art Gallery and Museum* was renamed for him and for his famous son: *The Wilson*. Yet still, most remember the son and know nothing of the father.

David Elder's fascinating book is the long overdue tonic to this, exploring as it does, the family, the life, the work and the achievements of Edward Thomas Wilson of Cheltenham.

Dr. David M. Wilson
Autumn 2021

Introduction

D R EDWARD THOMAS WILSON (1832-1918), known as ETW in family circles, was one of the great worthies of Cheltenham. As a medical practitioner during the Victorian and Edwardian periods he contributed greatly to the health and well-being of the town: he battled for clean drinking water, and pioneered innovations such as isolation fever hospitals and district nursing. However, his influence on the town he lived and worked in for nearly 60 years went much wider than the medical field alone; with a broad range of interests and expertise across both the arts and sciences, he was something of a 'Renaissance Man' figure in local circles. Establishing or contributing to various clubs and societies, including one of the country's oldest photographic societies, he also espoused numerous good causes - from helping to improve the living conditions of the poor to campaigning vigorously for the establishment of a free library, a museum and an art school. His legacy enriches the cultural life of the town to this day.

Spanning eighty-five years across the reign of four monarchs, his life also helps to illuminate some of the most significant scientific and socio-economic developments of his era. And through his family, he has direct links with two celebrated figures of the British Empire: his brother, Major-General Sir Charles William Wilson (1836-1905), led the doomed attempt to rescue General Gordon from Khartoum, and ETW shared his exasperation when he was scapegoated for the expedition's failure. As father of the Antarctic explorer, Dr Edward Adrian Wilson (1872-1912), who famously perished with Captain Scott at the South Pole, ETW was instrumental in encouraging his son's love of science, nature and exploration. Following news of the Polar tragedy, he also acted as the focal point for Cheltenham's grief.

This is the first biography of Edward Thomas Wilson, a deep-thinking man who declined fame and fortune in London hospitals to become a highly-regarded general practitioner and consultant in Cheltenham. It is hoped that through this volume his life and achievements will become more widely recognised and, perhaps also, inspire others to follow in the steps of a man whose epitaph reads, 'He went about doing good'.

Author's Note

THE MAIN PRIMARY SOURCE consulted for this biography is ETW's unpublished autobiography entitled *My Life* (referred to as *ML* in the notes). Covering the period until December 1916, his eighty-third birthday, the two-volume manuscript (and earlier draft volumes) are available for consultation by appointment at The Wilson, Cheltenham's art gallery and museum. For ease of reading and consistency of style, when quoting from this work I have made some minor presentational changes, for example replacing '+' with 'and'.

Acknowledgements

I WOULD LIKE TO ACKNOWLEDGE the considerable kindness of numerous individuals who have assisted in the production of this book in so many different ways. Particular thanks are due to Jill Barlow, Katie Barrett, Dr Steve Blake, John Chandler, Hannah Dale, Gary Davies, Sally Ferrers, Ian Gee, Ann-Rachael Harwood, James Hodsdon, Carrie Howse, Laura Ibbett, Saffron Mackay, Carly Manson, Katherine MacInnes, Anne Marcant, Rachael Merrison, Eric Miller, Dr Chris Morton, Geoff North, Dr Peter Ormerod, Sarah Pearson, Grace Pritchards Woods, Lindsay Raitt, Simon Rendall, Rachel Roberts, Benedict Sayers, Matthew Simpson, Anne Strathie, Élisabeth Venne, Jill Waller, John White, Eric Williams, and Alastair Wilson. My special thanks also to the Wilson family, in particular Dr David Wilson, for writing the foreword, commenting on the draft, and granting me permission (on behalf of the family) to access and make use of the family archive.

I am also particularly grateful to the support received from the following institutions (lately, because of the Covid pandemic, under difficult circumstances): The Wilson (Cheltenham Art Gallery and Museum); Cheltenham College Archives; Cheltenham Ladies' College Archives; Cheltenham Local Studies Library; Dean Close School; Gloucestershire Archives; St George's, University of London; The Thomas H. Manning Polar Archives, Scott Polar Research Institute, University of Cambridge; Royal College of Surgeons; Pitt Rivers Museum, University of Oxford; Friends in Council; and The Royal Archives, Windsor Castle.

I would also like to thank the following institutions and individuals who kindly supplied illustrations and/or granted permission to use them in this book: Cheltenham Borough Council and the Cheltenham Trust/The Wilson Family Collection for the images on pp. 4, 15, 18, 19, 26, 30, 36, 38, 41, 42, 49, 117, 131, 144, 167, 168, 191; Neela Mann for the images on pp. 188 (top and bottom), 207; David Hanks of Cotswold Images for the image on p. 75; Gary Davies for the images on pp. 3, 13; Geoff North for the image on p. 140; John White for the image on p. 254; Lindsay Raitt of Friends in Council for the images on pp. 50, 52, 169, 200; Brian Torode and Richard Barton for the image on p. 77; Cheltenham College Archives for the images on pp. 24 (bottom), 78, 103, 195; the Wellcome Collection for images on pp. 10, 14, 16, 57, 64, 71, 76, 93, 96, 153, 193; Library of Congress Archive for the images on pp. 29, 80, 135, 175, 187; Cheltenham Camera Club for the image on p. 34; Philadelphia Museum of Art: Gift of Theodore T. Newbold and Helen Cunningham, 2010, 2010-3-2 for the image on p. 39. Permission of Her Majesty Queen Elizabeth II has also been granted for the quotation from *Queen Victoria's Journal* (see p. 81).

Finally, my heartfelt thanks to my long-suffering family, Meg, Rachel and Catrin, for their patience, understanding and support.

1
Early Years (1832-59)

Birth and parentage – Hean Castle – School at St David's – Liverpool
Collegiate School – Oxford University – St George's Hospital – Paris

*'At the end of the bay to the left were rocks, honeycombed into caves – and in
these we revelled as children, climbing in and out giving free rein to our fancies
as to possible smugglers, or seals, or still more unlikely inhabitants. The rock
pools at extreme low water were lined with anenomies [sic] of most varied and
gorgeous hues. Indeed it would be difficult to meet with a spot more romantic
from its situation, or more suited for the bringing up of a young family with a
love for Nature in all her various moods ... '.*
~ ETW ~

ON SUNDAY 16 DECEMBER 1832 at 8 Wesley Street,[1] Princes Park,
Liverpool, the latest generation of a wealthy family that had made
its fortune in Liverpool and Philadelphia celebrated the winter birth of
their first son, Edward Thomas Wilson. The infant, who later developed
dark brown hair and grey blue eyes, became fondly known in the family
as ETW. The day was made even sweeter by the fact that the crying baby
had 'unconsciously won a bet'[2] by being born ahead of the first offspring of
friends who shared his parents' wedding anniversary. It was a happy end
to a year that had instilled much anxiety. Asiatic cholera, endemic to India,
had spread from the sub-continent causing severe diarrhoea, dehydration,
vomiting, and often death. Reaching Western Europe in 1831, it was
subsequently carried to North America aboard immigrant ships. By 1832
Liverpool and Philadelphia were particularly badly affected.

In Liverpool an epidemic in May and June led to nearly 5,000 cases,
about a third of which proved fatal. Members of the public became so
incensed about the authorities' inability to handle the crisis that a series
of disturbances broke out which became known as the Cholera Riots.
Crowds started to attack doctors and hospitals, fearing that some were
more interested in securing bodies for dissection than for cure. After all,
memories of the notorious activities of Burke and Hare in Edinburgh

in 1828 were still fresh in people's minds. In Philadelphia the death toll rose to around 930 as the disease ran its course by mid-September. One of the physicians who worked tirelessly to save lives in Philadelphia was ETW's uncle, Thomas Bellerby Wilson (1807-65), a quiet, shy, retiring, but immensely generous and knowledgeable man. During the summer of 1832, after recently qualifying in medicine and then acquiring experience of the epidemics in Europe, Thomas devoted his services gratuitously to one of the city's hospitals for the poor rather than establish a lucrative medical practice for himself. By the autumn he had to leave the city to restore his own health.

Although the Wilsons on both sides of the Atlantic escaped the scourge of cholera at that time, they remained anxious about this frightening disease given the confusion that persisted about cholera outbreaks. It was not until the middle of the nineteenth century that the pioneers of modern epidemiology started to gain a clearer understanding about how the disease was originally transmitted and how it could be contained and treated. John Snow's study in 1854, which identified the cause of the London cholera outbreak in Soho, was particularly ground-breaking. Little did ETW's parents think then that, years later, their child would also become a pioneer in modern epidemiology and the fight against infectious diseases, initially following in the footsteps of his uncle Thomas through becoming a qualified physician.

Thomas Bellerby was just one of the many interesting and colourful characters within the family into which ETW had now been born. On his father's side the family stretched back into ancient Westmorland and descended from a long line of Quakers, although there had not been a Quaker in direct descent for two generations by the time he was born. The last had been his grandfather, Edward Wilson of Liverpool and Philadelphia (1772-1843), who established a fortune through land in America, the birth of the railways, and investments in the Philadelphia-Liverpool iron trade. He was a friend of George Stephenson, of 'Rocket' fame, and one of the few people to successfully reclaim lands in the United States after the War of Independence. The children inherited fortunes, and the sons styled themselves 'gentlemen'; they were inveterate collectors and were major benefactors of public institutions on more than one continent. Edward Wilson of Hean Castle (1808-88), ETW's father (see Appendix 1 for his family tree), was one of these. He brought together what was reputed to be

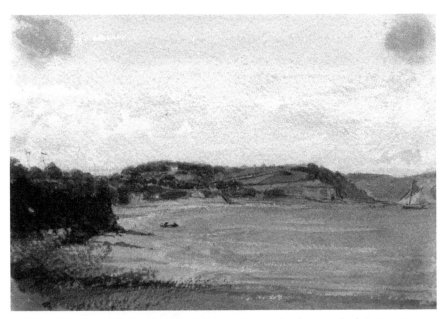

Hean Castle, visible on the hill, with Saundersfoot harbour to the left. Painting by Dorothy Jane Harvey, c.1860s.

the finest collection of hummingbirds in existence, and the Wilson's bird-of-paradise (*Cicinnurus respublica*) was named after him. He became High Sheriff of Pembrokeshire in 1861 and was a widely respected landowner. However, at the time of ETW's birth he worked for the firm of merchant bankers, Brown, Shipley & Company.[3]

On his mother's side the Stokes family, whose motto *Fortis qui insons* means 'Strong is the innocent', inherited the large estate of Hean Castle[4] in Pembrokeshire following ETW's maternal grandfather's marriage into the Wogan family. This long-established family traced its descent from Sir John Wogan, who became chief justice and governor of Ireland during the time of Edward I. Susannah Wogan, ETW's grandmother, was the estate's co-heiress with her sister Eleanor. In 1800 she agreed to buy Eleanor's share for £7,200. ETW's mother, Frances Stokes (1812-91), known as Fanny, was one of Susannah's seven daughters, all noted beauties with raven black hair and dark brown eyes. Fanny was remembered in particular for a quick temper, a tendency to be 'excessively tidy', and her enjoyment of riding, needlework and art, for which she had a fair talent.[5]

Although the Wilsons in Liverpool survived the cholera pandemic during the 1830s, infant mortality was still an all-too-common threat.

William Henry, a younger brother for ETW, was born on 11 October 1834, but he quickly succumbed to inflammation of the lungs and died within three months. Nevertheless, another brother, Charles William, was more fortunate. Born on 14 March 1836, he would become one of ETW's closest siblings.

Aged just three, ETW started school in September 1836 – at a small private establishment run by one Anne Davidson. While one of his earliest memories was the sight of children's excited faces when they saw sticklebacks swimming about inside a bottle acquired by local street urchins, his most vivid memory was related to disease: the scarred face of a female servant, who worked at the school, her disfigurement the result of smallpox.

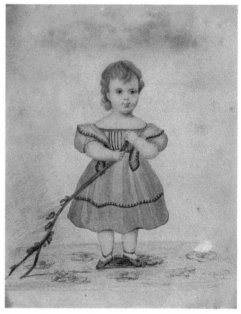

Portrait of ETW as a young child

The spectre of smallpox continued to lurk during his early years. A new epidemic swept through the country from the south-west, claiming 42,000 lives in England and Wales from July 1837 to December 1840. Shortly after the death of William IV on 20 June 1837 – a day when ETW recalled the newspapers being printed with black mourning borders - Fanny unwittingly took her two sons into the epicentre of the outbreak as she re-settled the family temporarily at the Stokes' family home at Hean Castle. ETW's father had decided to try his hand in the colliery business, going into partnership with his father-in-law, Thomas Stokes, whose son he came to know through Brown, Shipley & Company. Fanny initially took the children to Hean Castle, so that their father could join them once the house in Liverpool could be vacated. They then travelled a further 8 miles from Hean Castle to their new residence at Lydstep House (now converted into a holiday park restaurant), approximately 4 miles from Tenby. Although they had all been vaccinated against smallpox, Fanny contracted the disease almost immediately after arriving in Pembrokeshire and infected the other members of the household. Despite this, while ETW's aunt Emily showed severe symptoms and became badly pockmarked, the rest of the family had a fortunate escape.

In Pembrokeshire, the family settled into a new way of life, surrounded by the natural world in all its infinite variety. Their two-storey house was practically on the beach, separated from the sea by only a high pebble ridge. Behind it rose the steep limestone cliffs of Lydstep Haven. Outside the house, a monkey which the family kept as a pet used to frighten away tramps. Opposite, looking out of the bay towards the south-east was Caldey Island. Lying just 4 miles away, this became a favourite destination for ETW and Charly, as ETW called his brother. The two would often venture there in their father's boat to see puffin, shelduck, chough and peregrine and to look for items to add to the natural history collections of birds' eggs, crabs, and flowers that their father encouraged them to keep. Sometimes they brought home guillemot eggs – not for the collection, but for the family table. There were occasionally problems with rats, dealt with by ETW's father who chased them through the house, wielding a poker in one hand. At Lydstep House, the Wilson family grew. The brothers gained two sisters, Elizabeth Ann (b. 1838) and Fanny Georgina (b. 1841).

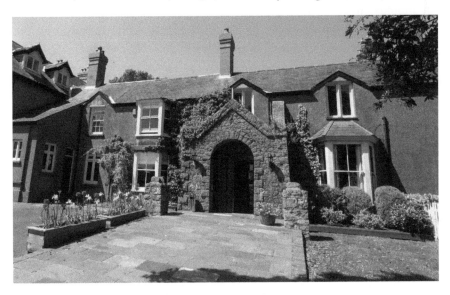

Lydstep House today

The area provided ETW with a wild, open adventure playground. The boys went bathing and fishing, played imaginary smuggling games in caves, and learned how to scull a boat with a single oar. However, they avoided venturing too close to the neighbouring quicksand in case they got caught and swallowed up in it. ETW developed a special interest in the marine flora and fauna, marvelling in particular at the myriad colours and hues of the anemones that he found in the rock pools at low tide. At a very early age, when just eight years old, he also learned how to shoot after his father gave him a small single-barrelled gun. Stalking through the surrounding countryside, he went to hunt not just rabbit, but also polecat, woodcock, snipe, golden plover, and, on one occasion, a rare glaucous gull which visited the bay. His passion for hunting was so strong that it continued as a favourite pastime well into his late seventies. Although life at Lydstep was undoubtedly 'wild and free', ETW later recognised that it had the disadvantage of making them rather 'shy and retiring'.[6]

The sea naturally formed an important part in their lives. On the one hand, it could be threatening, with high spring tides sometimes reaching the boundaries of the house, and on one occasion even penetrating into the cellar - ETW's father nearly drowned as he tried to pump out the invading sea water. On the other hand, the sea brought much-needed contact with the outside world, with numerous ships from Devon, Cornwall, Cardigan and Ireland arriving into Lydstep Haven to transport limestone from the local quarries. This allowed ETW to befriend some of the ships' captains. Following a request from his father, one was even so obliging as to extract and carry over some limestone pavement from the Giant's Causeway, which was subsequently used to ornament the garden of Lydstep House.[7]

The sea also brought ETW closer to the outside world in other ways. At the age of eight he attended the Cathedral School at St. David's, the first part of the journey being by boat to Milford Haven. Unfortunately, life in this new world began unhappily. The Reverend Nathaniel Davies, the school's headmaster, had a later reputation as a cruel, tyrannical taskmaster, and whilst the teaching could be described as 'mechanical but good' it was also 'driven into [them] at the point of the cane'.[8] Birching on bare hands was administered hourly every day and no-one escaped the punishment since it was given for no other reason than to inculcate obedience. Anyone who committed a proper offence was dealt with even more severely. A boy arriving at school in wet boots, for example, was beaten mercilessly on the soles of his feet to act as a deterrent for others. The general atmosphere engendered there was one of 'sink or swim' - almost literally so when sea-bathing sessions took place. ETW commented:

> Bathing in these early years was a torture. The small boys were hunted out from their hiding places, driven like slaves to the shore and made to undress in a cave with the headmaster. He could not swim himself but he delighted in taking us out beyond our depths and letting us struggle in as we could.[9]

At least school life led to the formation of new friendships and acquaintances, among whom, ETW recalled, was Lewis Morris (1833-1907) who became a well-known Welsh poet and politician. Although the boys' unhappiness at St David's never translated into outright rebellion, more generally there was protest in the air. Between 1839 and 1843 tensions were rising in South Wales. At night time ETW would sometimes hear the distant sound of horns blowing from the surrounding hillside farms as agricultural workers expressed their dissatisfaction with high levels of taxation. Later on, squads of soldiers were quartered in St David's. They had been sent to keep an eye on the participants of what later became known as the Rebecca Riots. As the soldiers looked for ways to occupy their time it also became an opportunity for ETW to witness the soldiers practising the remarkable trick of shooting a tallow candle through a wooden door (quite possible if using a musket).

Around this time there were further additions to the family. In 1844, when ETW was eleven, a second brother Henry Josiah (known as Harry) was born and then, two years later, Rathmel George, his youngest brother, arrived. Given the age differences, however, ETW spent most time with his eldest brother Charly who joined him at the Cathedral School in 1844. Then, a year later, both were liberated from St David's, going north to Liverpool to continue their education at the city's new Collegiate Institution (surviving today as Liverpool College). Originally opened by William Gladstone only two years earlier, the Ciceronian motto of the college, *Non solum ingenii verum etiam virtutis*, means 'Not only the intellect but also the character'. Despite the college's intent to educate the whole person, ETW found the teaching left much to be desired. The standards and targets were generally dictated according to social class: the upper school, for example, was reserved for those destined for university; the middle school for an 'upper class commercial education'; and the lower school for 'the trading classes'.[10] Much to ETW's disappointment, he ended up in what was dubbed the 'dunce's class' and consequently learned very little.[11] Although university exhibitions were available through which boys could climb from the bottom to the top, unfortunately for ETW, competition for these was fierce. In his case he was narrowly beaten by John Rigby (1834-1903) who later achieved recognition as the Attorney General and the Lord Justice of Appeal. Despite some teaching deficiencies, ETW enjoyed many aspects of school life: there was the inspiring location of the school, overlooking the mouth of the River Mersey and conveniently close to the famous Everton toffee shop, which frequently took toll of his pocket money. Boys also had the chance to witness outstanding performances in the school hall, among them several by the 'Swedish Nightingale', the highly acclaimed opera singer Jenny Lind (1820-87).

ETW remained in Liverpool from 1845 to 1851. During the long summer and winter holidays, he would often return home to Pembrokeshire, travelling there via Bristol. In the days before the Clifton suspension bridge the journey was challenging, even for the intrepid. After arriving in Bristol, passengers transferred into a basket, which was then hauled across the Avon gorge by ropes, the more nervous travellers probably choosing not to peer into the chasm below. An alternative option - by coach, rowing boat and steamer - involved at least twenty hours simply for the sea journey between Milford Haven and Liverpool. To ward off sea-sickness on this voyage ETW would often turn to a bottle of 'excellent milk punch',[12] as recommended by his doctor.

ETW spent some holiday time away from home. His father occasionally encouraged his sons to go away on their own for long walking, fishing and hunting expeditions. With little money but plenty of encouragement to make their limited funds last as long as possible, they were charged with giving a detailed account when they returned of everything they had seen and done. Cicero would have approved. If there was a single experience that helped ETW to develop a well-rounded character, this was the one he found of greatest value. It was also one he would later pass on to his own offspring.

There were also regular visits to ETW's relatives in Liverpool, among whom was his kind though 'somewhat formidable' Aunt Susan who was always dressed in her stiff Quaker costume.[13] It was through Susan that ETW came to know her brother Francis Frith (1822-98), the Victorian pioneer of travel photography. Additionally, there were visits with his father - to the Lake District, Knowsley and also, in 1847, to London where his father was engaged in adding to his unique collection of hummingbirds. Equally interesting was life back home in Pembrokeshire. There were parties at Tenby and formal balls at Pembroke, where the Wilsons rubbed shoulders with the elite of the county, whilst at Lydstep House itself the drawing-room was filled with inspiring tales of adventure. One of the most memorable occurred in 1848 during a visit by ETW's Uncle William. Following the overthrow of King Louis Philippe, revolution had broken out in Paris, leading the family to be concerned for the safety of ETW's aunt and young family who resided there at the time. His father and uncle immediately rushed off to the French capital where they arrived just in time, not only to ensure the safety of the stricken family members, but also to witness piles of books from the Royal Library being set alight in the courtyard of the Tuileries Palace. ETW noted 'We had some of the leaves [from the Royal Library books] for many years which were rescued and brought home as curios'.[14]

Soon, it would be time for the two brothers to decide on their own paths of adventure. For Charly, it was a straightforward matter. Having already set his mind on a military career he left Liverpool in 1852 at the age of sixteen to continue his studies at Cheltenham College with its well-established military tradition. For ETW, however, there was less certainty about the path to be followed and, for the time being, he decided to continue his education at university. In May 1851, he matriculated at Exeter College, Oxford.

In the 1850s, Oxford was a relatively small city. Largely contained within its medieval boundaries, the population comprised approximately 28,000, of which the university constituted about 5 or 6 per cent. ETW took a little while to settle into his new surroundings. His accommodation in the attic of a corner staircase overlooking Broad Street was so cramped that he had to sit on the foot of the bed to wash. The atmosphere at Exeter College around this time was described as 'quiet, gentlemanlike, and decorous, though a little slow'.[15] He found the first term at Oxford 'somewhat dull' given that most of his friends had gone to Cambridge.[16] Moreover, he was made to feel inferior by the rather aloof Exeter men who

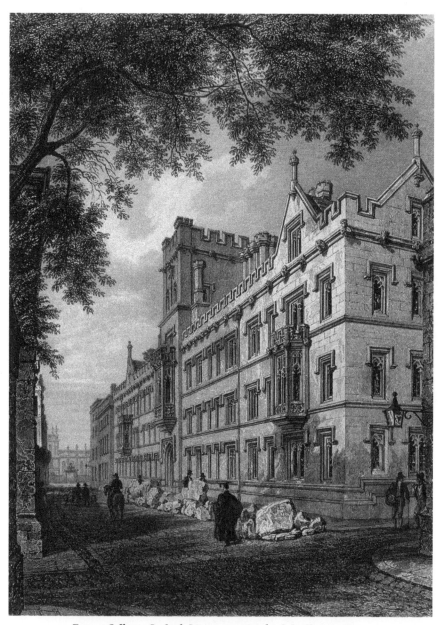

Exeter College, Oxford. Line engraving by J. Le Keux, 1835,
after F. Mackenzie.

rated their fellows largely on whether they had rowed at Eton or played
cricket at Harrow or Winchester. Despite this, he soon made close friends,
among whom were Charles Cave (1832-1922), later a successful banker

who became knighted after serving in several offices, including as High Sheriff of Bristol and of Devon, and Philip Sclater (1829-1913) who, after studying Law at Corpus Christi College, became an expert ornithologist and Secretary of the Zoological Society of London.

ETW took up rowing as one of his main recreational pursuits and soon became caught up in the thrill and excitement of the annual series of bumping races known as the Torpids. In those days, training for the boat races was far from scientific. Although smoking and drinking wine were eschewed, the exercise itself merely consisted of a jog around Christ Church meadow after a practice row. ETW's diet largely consisted of raw chop or steak with a limited amount of vegetables and beer. It usually left him in a poor state for rowing for hours after a meal. In one race, he nearly collapsed after winning the first heat whilst, in another, he unavoidably threw up before lifting the winners' cup. He also noted wryly that a 'whole mould of jelly per man after the race was scarcely conducive to work next day.'[17] While on the river, ETW would occasionally see Henry Kingsley (1830-76), the novelist and brother of Charles Kingsley (1819-75), rowing daily on the river and carrying the unfortunate reputation as 'the ugliest man in Oxford'.[18] Rowing also allowed ETW to explore and venture further afield. During periods of flood, he would row for miles over the drowned meadows, charging the gaps in the fences but also, on one winter's day, having to swim for the bank whilst wearing a thick coat after his boat capsized. Rowing brought enjoyable social events too; there were boat suppers, usually attended by thirty or forty students at a time - with drinks, smoking and games of cards. During his term of residence (1851-54) at Exeter College, ETW noticed a curious change in smoking habits:

> ... on my first going a pipe was considered quite out of place and was seen only in private rooms and then only rarely. Cigars were de rigeur – yet before I left ... a pipe was "the thing" and cigars fit for only "the Master".[19]

On the academic side, teaching standards at Exeter College were variable: there was a 'cold, unsympathetic teacher of Aristotle', who was in the habit of stopping his lectures promptly just as the hour struck, not even bothering to finish the sentence, and then resuming next time at the precise word which had ended the last lecture.[20] Unsurprisingly, ETW found the lectures of the extra-collegiate professors of greater interest. Among these was Dr Charles Daubeny (1795–1867) who, whilst being a brilliant chemist, created much amusement by conducting laborious experiments which invariably went wrong. Once, ETW recorded, when 'a bottle was passed round the class with a warning not to open it as it was offensive, an overpowering vapour would soon be apparent coming from the back benches – and would set everyone coughing or render the room untenable'.[21] Oxford also brought other opportunities: while visiting Dr Henry Acland (1815-1900), the famous physician who introduced the study of natural science into Oxford University, ETW met John Ruskin (1819-1900), one of the greatest figures of the Victorian age. Initially, Ruskin had been engrossed with Acland, admiring the fall of light on some green leaves in the garden's summer house.

Whilst applying himself fully to his studies, ETW also looked forward greatly to the summer terms at Oxford: then, serious reading gave way to more relaxed punting on the River Cherwell, and a constant stream of balls and garden fêtes at which there was 'ample opportunity for flirtation and occasionally for more serious love-making'.[22]

By the time ETW returned home to Pembrokeshire in the summer of 1852, it was to Hean Castle rather than Lydstep House that he travelled since, by then, ETW's father had purchased Hean Castle from his brother-in-law, Thomas Stokes. It was not until 21 June 1854 that the Wilson family took full possession of it when the local press reported: 'At four o'clock in the afternoon the cannons [at Saundersfoot] commenced firing, and the bells ringing merrily, which were kept up with intense ardour until a late hour'; then, the family was 'met by a large and respectable company of tenants and neighbours, bearing banners' and welcomed with 'cheering and rejoicings of multitudes, where [Edward Wilson, Esq.] regaled them with plenty of strong ale. After which each member returned to his respective home highly gratified'.[23] The mansion[24] and 700-acre estate comprised rich meadows, pasture, arable and woodland, and included sea frontage of 1¼ miles in length. There was good fishing in the neighbourhood, and the woodcock hunting was reputedly second to none. Its value was further enhanced by the wealth of its minerals which included anthracite coal, iron ore and fire clay. There was also the added advantage that these could be easily exploited through their proximity to Saundersfoot harbour, without damaging the picturesque landscape.

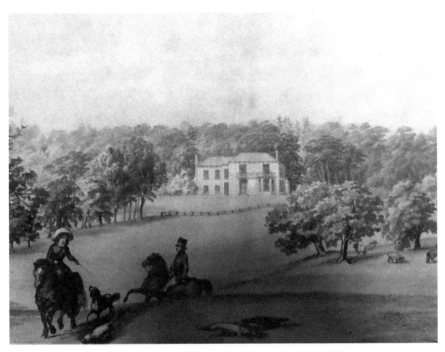

Hean Castle. Print taken from an 1850s sales brochure.

Whilst the memories of her childhood home were happily rekindled here for ETW's mother, the challenge of running a new business venture now firmly lay upon the shoulders of ETW's father.

After settling into the new family home, ETW then decided to undertake a long expedition, alone, through France and parts of Switzerland and Belgium. During this trip, he once walked 42 miles in a day, with a knapsack, over the Grimsel and Furka mountain passes in the Swiss Alps - reaching elevations over approximately 7,900 feet. Arriving back in London shortly after 14 September, however, he was surprised to see flags at half-mast along the River Thames. Field Marshal Arthur Wellesley, the First Duke of Wellington (1769-1852) had just died. ETW immediately rushed back to Oxford to obtain leave so that he could see at first hand the body lying in state at Chelsea Hospital. It was the most solemnly impressive sight he had ever witnessed. He commented:

> the silence and the gloom, the Guardsmen with reversed arms, the body of the old warrior ... everything tended to touch the deepest chords of feeling and awe.[25]

In 1853 ETW paid his first visit to Cheltenham where he saw Charly, still at Cheltenham College, and his sisters Elizabeth and Fanny who were staying at Miss Smee's ten-bedroomed house[26] in Bayshill Road. The two brothers proceeded to go on a holiday to Ireland, ETW returning later after touring further through Scotland and the Lakes. In the following May, ETW successfully passed his Classical Exam (or First Final) at Oxford. For his Second Final, he now had to choose between mathematics, history and law, or natural science (the 'Stinks'). Choosing the latter on account of his passion for natural history, he was soon engrossed in the dissection of worms, snails and newts. He attended lectures at the Christ Church Museum, encountering amusing tales of the theologian and geologist Dean William Buckland (1784-1856), which had entered the museum's folklore. On one occasion, ETW heard, Buckland had obtained an alligator for one of the dissection classes, and then, 'in the interests of science', distributed steaks from the animal to the dons. Perhaps not surprisingly, the college became 'much disturbed throughout the night'.[27]

ETW also visited London to prepare for his natural science exam, working in Carey Street in the laboratory of the eminent microscopist Dr Lionel Beale (1828-1906). During this time, he made careful studies

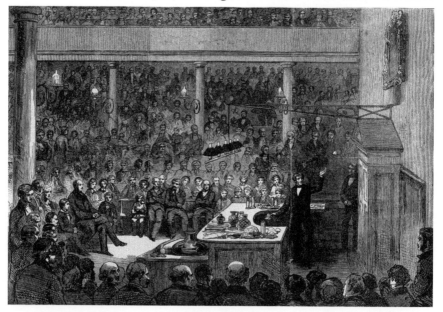

Michael Faraday lecturing at the Royal Institution. Wood engraving, 1856, after A. Blaikley.

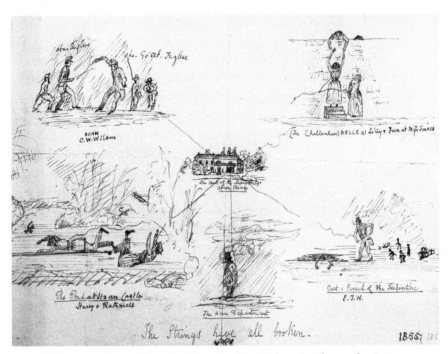

'The strings have all broken'. Drawing by a Wilson family member, 1855

of skeletons at both the Museum of the Royal College of Surgeons and the British Museum. He attended lectures at the Royal Institution, once sitting next to Dr David Livingstone (1813-73), whom he described as 'a most attentive listener'.[28] On another occasion, attending a lecture in front of the Prince Consort, he heard Michael Faraday (1791-1867) give a presentation on electricity. He found Faraday's coolness and perseverance in repeating a delicate experiment over and over again until it finally succeeded highly inspirational.[29]

During his final term at Oxford in May 1855, building work on the New Museum (later to become Oxford University Museum of Natural History) was nearing completion. ETW's father donated a column of Lydstep marble, which still adorns one of the galleries, serving to illustrate the phase of grey limestone during one of the geological periods. ETW himself helped launch an appeal to raise money for statues of Aristotle and the French naturalist Georges Cuvier (1769-1832). ETW's preparatory work in London paid off, and he gained a First Class in Natural Science.

By now, the family's apron strings had certainly been stretched, if not 'broken'. While dark clouds ominously gather over 'The Home

Department', Elizabeth and Fanny appear to be enjoying secretive adventures at Miss Smee's lodgings. The humorous sketch also depicts Harry and Rathmel taking a tumble on the frozen Hean Castle estate pond, while Charly, then residing at Bonn University, where he was improving his modern languages, is engaged in his military career. Yet, what next for ETW who appears smoking his pipe while skating on thin ice on the Serpentine in London? Although, like his brother, ETW also considered joining the army, in a time of relative peace, he thought, this option would lead to 'an idle life'.[30] He quickly discounted law, which he disliked, but was somewhat attracted to the church. In the end, after consulting Dr Henry Acland, Regius Professor of Medicine at Oxford, he decided on medicine. This was partly out of personal preference, but there was also a practical point: he had already completed much of the required work in anatomy and physiology. Therefore, on 1 October 1855 he entered St George's Hospital, London, as a physician student.

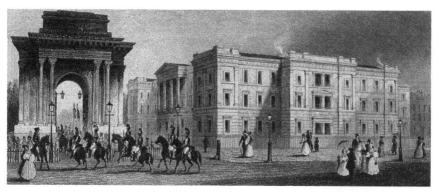

St George's Hospital and the Constitution Arch, Hyde Park Corner.

The hospital was then at Hyde Park Corner. Twice a day ETW walked there from his lodgings above a haberdasher's shop at 34 Upper Seymour Street – a pleasant walk through Hyde Park. Later, he reflected:

> I made the fatal mistake, as things turned out, of aiming at the higher branches of the profession without going through the drudgery of the lower. Never feeling certain what I should practice I took the course which took my fancy rather than that which could equip me for the actual requirements of a medical life.[31]

Although it was an exciting time to be embarking on a course in medicine, ETW was to find that not all lecturers were open to the latest advances. His lecturer on clinical medicine despised the new-fangled invention of the stethoscope, preferring to place his ear on the patient's back. 'Of real teaching, there was very little', ETW commented, and he considered his own work 'more or less dilettante' because, as heir to the vast fortune at Hean Castle, he never expected to have to earn a living through his chosen profession.[32]

During the holidays, ETW continued to enjoy carefree days at Hean Castle. The Lydstep Haven coast made for exciting, though sometimes dangerous, times as he played with his younger brothers Harry and Rathmel. Watched over by the local quarrymen, the three would dive from a large rock into the raging water below, with many jagged boulders lying hidden just beneath the surface. In stormy conditions, they were sometimes forced to swim nearly a mile to reach the safety of the shore, often encountering swarms of jellyfish, shoals of mackerel or the occasional porpoise. Once, when they met a shoal of jellyfish, the brothers started throwing them at each other until one hit ETW in the eye, causing him to reel in agony as the sting inflamed his eye.

Life in London was not all study. On 29 May 1856 ETW witnessed the poignant return of troops from the Crimean War in Hyde Park where the force from the crowds was enough to lift him off the ground for 50 yards. He also visited Chatham to see Charly, now a Commissioned Lieutenant in the Royal Engineers, and made a further visit to see him on 31 March 1858, immediately prior to Charly's departure to British Columbia. For the next four years, as Secretary and Transport Officer of the North American Boundary Commission, Charly's task was to mark the line of the 49th parallel from the Rocky Mountains to the Pacific Ocean. Here, he would have to contend with the extreme climate and (in some places) the danger of rattlesnakes.

With his Bachelor of Medicine examination at Oxford soon approaching, ETW decided to brush up his medical botany with his friend William Ogle[33] by visiting Kew Gardens, where they had been granted privileged morning access by Sir Joseph Hooker (1817-1911). They were regularly greeted in the mornings by the gardening enthusiast Princess Mary Adelaide of Cambridge (1833-97), later the Duchess of Teck. The extra preparations paid off, and ETW passed his medical exams on 17

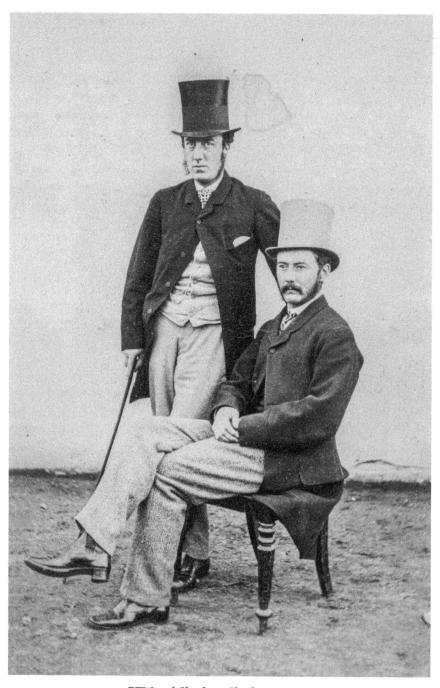

ETW and Charly at Chatham, 1858

June. Returning home for a pleasant summer, at that time there was no sign of impending problems in the fortunes of the Hean Castle Estate. ETW then travelled to Paris with William Ogle to learn about some of the latest developments and thinking in modern medical practices during the winter session. As they crossed the English Channel on the night of 15 October the two friends witnessed the spectacle of Donati's comet lighting up the sky. ETW noted that Arcturus was shining clearly through the comet's tail.[34]

Having taken lodgings in the Latin Quarter, they rose early every morning to arrive at the Hôtel-Dieu hospital before breakfast. Here, they heard lectures from the eminent physician Armand Trousseau (1801-67) who was then focussing on the treatment of diphtheria. Trousseau was the first physician in France to perform a tracheotomy, using this procedure to open the airways in some of his diphtheria patients. Just how successful Trousseau's approach ultimately was, ETW thought, was difficult to judge. While he praised Trousseau's lectures as 'oratorical triumphs', in hindsight he felt that some of his methods left much to be desired: in particular, he noticed that his patients were left at risk of contracting other diseases: smallpox cases were usually close to others suffering from tuberculosis or pneumonia.[35]

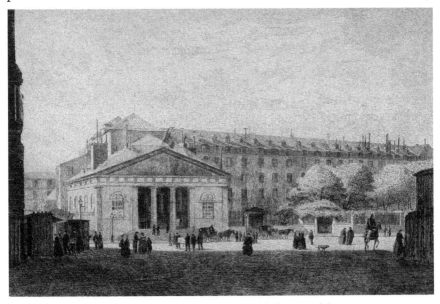

The Hôtel Dieu, Paris. Etching, possibly by Grimdel, 1877

Other treatments that they witnessed might have been inspired by a handbook of torture from the Middle Ages. They came across a ward full of hysterical women who were being treated through the placement of red-hot irons on their abdomens. 'Strange to say', thought ETW, 'after the alarm of the first application no objection was made or serious pain complained of'. He further opined that it 'probably was a very efficient remedy for a limited number of cases'.[36] On other occasions, it was clear to ETW that many of the innovative experiments being tested were doomed to fail. At the Hôpital de la Charité, he witnessed the early experiments in electrical painless dentistry, using street urchins as subjects. The procedure involved giving an electric shock just before the tooth was extracted. As ETW noted, there was invariably a loud scream from the victim; and although the dentist tried to persuade the audience that there had been no pain, one of the surgeons came forward and, after questioning the boy, announced, '"Messieurs il a suffert diablement."'.[37] After that, ETW recorded, nothing more was heard of electrical dentistry. Another visit they made was to the celebrated Abattoirs de Grenelle (or Abattoirs des Invalides) where, ETW was shocked to witness, not only butchery on an industrial scale, but also a soldier sitting up to his neck in a tub of warm coagulated blood. At the time, this was thought to be an effective remedy for rheumatism but, as with electrical dentistry, this treatment was subsequently abandoned.

Despite these oddities, the two friends were still greatly inspired by their exposure to some successful new ideas and approaches. They heard, for example, interesting and informative lectures, including one from the Mauritian physiologist Charles-Édouard Brown-Séquard (1817-94) on the recent discovery of glycogen in the liver. Moreover, they met several highly-regarded physicians, including Auguste Nélaton (1807-73), later the personal surgeon of Napoleon III, and the eminent French zoologist Henri Milne-Edwards (1800-85). They also witnessed several new important developments, such as experiments on the stimulation of nerves and muscles using electric current, conducted by Guillaume-Benjamin-Amand Duchenne (1806-75) who, later, became recognised as the inventor of electrotherapy. Equally impressive were the rhinoplasty operations they observed. These were commonly performed at the Hôtel-Dieu, using transplanted healthy skin to restore deficiencies in noses affected by disease or accident.

The Paris experience also encouraged them to challenge their own beliefs and preconceptions: ETW was particularly fascinated with the routine use in France of tisanes or herbal infusions, which led to positive recovery rates for patients. He was also struck by the French doctors' overzealous use of surgery, observing that 'we preferred the caution of a Caesar Hawkins or a Brodie' – two surgeons who both favoured trying to save limbs wherever possible.[38] The trip also challenged ETW's moral conscience after he observed vivisection for the first time. As a lover of nature, he had serious doubts about the ethics involved in the practice but, on balance, considered that the ends did justify the means as long as it could be carefully planned and controlled. He commented:

> It was unpleasant, painful – but if man is of more value than many sparrows, if he is justified in killing for his food, in killing to rid himself of an enemy or pest; or for his mere amusement in sport; then it is clear to me that well planned careful experiments on animals with a view to the alleviation of suffering and disease are not only justifiable but meritorious.[39]

Paris at this time under Napoleon III was particularly lively. The two friends revelled in the frequent reviews of the troops whose vibrant uniforms brightened up the overcast days of winter. Occasionally, they caught sight of the carriage carrying the Emperor, the Empress and the young Prince Imperial, as it drove past. On the cultural side, ETW's interest in art was stimulated by frequent visits to the Louvre, while his musical senses were heightened by magnificent carol-singing on Christmas Eve from members of the Opera at one of the local churches.

On New Year's Day in 1859 came the thrill of the Bal Masqué at the Paris Opera. Shortly after, and quite out of the blue, ETW received a letter inviting him to become a lecturer in Natural Sciences at Exeter College, Oxford, if a fellowship could be created. Unfortunately, the fellowship never materialised. Rather dejectedly, therefore, he returned to Hean Castle where, during the spring, he indulged his passion for exploring and collecting the flora and fauna of the Pembrokeshire coast. 'I never tired', he commented, 'of hunting on the sands and shores and on the land for flowers which grew in great profusion – many of them rare'.[40] He also took the opportunity to visit some old school friends, the Fothergills, who owned the Taff Vale iron-works.[41] Here, ETW marvelled at how the pigs of iron were formed after the furnaces were 'drawn', a stream of molten iron filling the moulds. From the Fothergills' bedroom window, he watched in awe as the solid blocks of glowing iron were continuously being fashioned into miles of railway track day and night.

While production soared in this part of the South Wales valleys, ETW soon discovered how different the fortunes of the colliery business were in Pembrokeshire, at Hean Castle. There seemed no reason for the family business to fail. The estate's natural resources were highly prized. ETW's father, mother and sisters were all well liked. His father helped to repair St Issel's, the parish church of Saundersfoot, and improved the cottages for the poorer tenants, while the rest of the family had provided other assistance, including teaching the poor in local schools. Yet, the business started to falter. As Wilson family folklore records, ETW and Charly were summoned into their father's study. Unaware of the reasons why, they heard him gravely tell them they would now both need to work for a living.

2
Cheltenham (1859-64)

Appointed Physician at Cheltenham General Hospital – Mary Agnes
Whishaw – Sanitary Statistics

*'Cheltenham was gay then, and as a bachelor one was asked everywhere. I
was never tired; a run of two to three miles before breakfast, Dispensary work
in the morning with visits in various parts of the town, for I always followed
up my patients to their homes, then a long walk or a row to Upton in the
afternoon, a dinner party, and possibly a dance to wind up, where I might
be found merrily engaged in a polka or galop towards the early hours of the
following day'.*
~ ETW ~

O N 23 AUGUST 1859 ETW set off on horseback from Hean Castle
aiming to meet a coach that would take him to Cheltenham. Earlier,
supported by glowing testimonials, he had successfully applied for the
post of Physician at the General Hospital and Dispensary in the attractive
Regency town. Describing him as 'an industrious, exemplary student',
'a thorough gentleman, of a very kind disposition', and someone who is
'earnest, painstaking, and loves his profession', ETW's testimonials also
suggested that he would 'discharge the most responsible duties of his
profession with honour, ability and kindness'.[1]

Unfortunately, the day got off to an inauspicious start. He was late
meeting the coach, and so pushed his horse hard to catch up with the
coach that was speeding ahead with his luggage. Suddenly, disaster struck;
the mare fell awkwardly, breaking her front knees. ETW tumbled to the
ground, damaging his right shoulder and narrowly escaping more serious
injury. Despite this misfortune, he eventually got to Cheltenham and was
still able to begin his medical duties straight away. From the outset, he
found the work stimulating at the Branch Dispensary and was impressed
by his colleagues, particularly Dr John Abercrombie (1817-92), whom he
quickly befriended. Like ETW, Dr Abercrombie had studied at St George's
and shared a similar temperament to him, being described as 'modest and
retiring' and 'content to live a quietly useful and an honourable life'.[2]

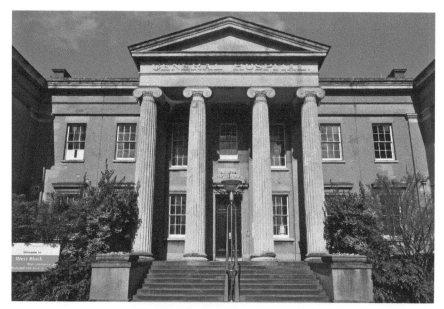

Cheltenham General Hospital today

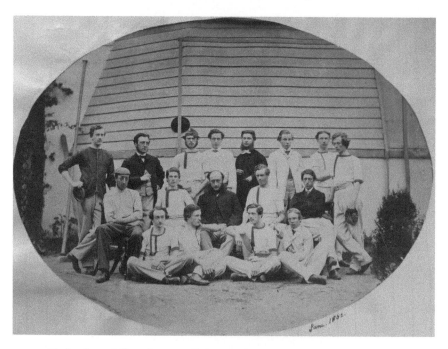

Cheltenham College Rowing Club 1862 (ETW is standing second on left)

Taking lodgings at 28 (now 55) Montpellier Terrace, ETW settled into the town quickly and made many new friends, particularly among a convivial group of Cheltenham College masters. It was with these College friendships that ETW started to share his Oxford passion for rowing, and soon helped set up the Cheltenham College Boat Club. Members of the club were only admitted if their achievements so warranted it, with the hope that they would 'stimulate others by their example of self-denial and manly desire to excel, to maintain the high character of [the] body, and be ever watchful for its welfare and its interests'.[3]

ETW also accompanied the College masters and boys on daily runs across the Shurdington fields, a routine which helped him achieve the feat of running a mile in under five minutes. Another favourite sport during his early years at Cheltenham was boxing, although this caused considerable consternation to his domestic servant who was certain that the house was being demolished during bouts.

Despite making a positive start in employment, ETW suffered a slight setback in November when he contracted scarlet fever from the children of one of his patients. Prevailing medical thinking was that the disease might be caused by an excess of blood. Without any more effective treatments available, his doctor prescribed leeches, and while ETW took this in his stride, he never forgot the horror on the face of his domestic servant when she was instructed to apply the segmented worms to his gums.

Apart from work and sport there was a whirlwind of social activity for ETW to enjoy in the town. Cheltenham's proximity to Oxford allowed him to keep in touch with friends from Exeter College days, one of whom encouraged him to apply for the post of Physician at the Radcliffe Infirmary. However, he dismissed the idea – reluctantly, in retrospect – since he was just settling into Cheltenham. If staying in Cheltenham had set some limits on his medical career, he was in no doubt that remaining there had brought with it many other advantages. Among these was his acquaintance with Mary Agnes Whishaw (1841-1930), the pretty daughter of a retired Russian merchant who was living at Keynsham House, at the eastern end of town. Seeing her at a party in conversation with some friends, ETW was immediately struck by her beauty, not least her greenish-grey eyes and the light brown locks of her hair which were tinged with gold. Her personality was equally attractive, marked by an energetic and forthright nature. ETW had fallen in love. His feelings for

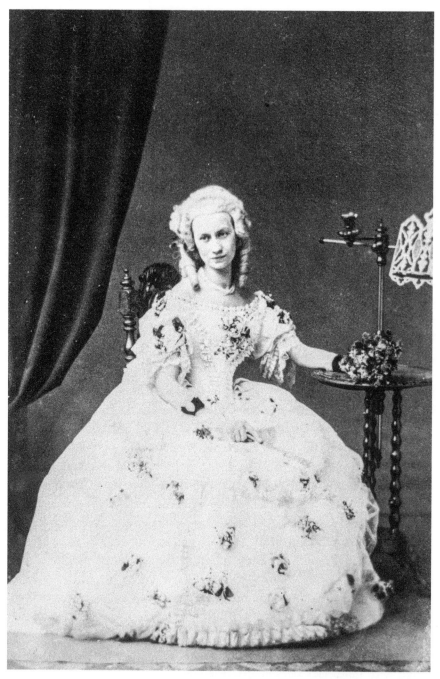

M. A. Whishaw (possibly dressed for a private theatrical).

Mary were greatly encouraged when he was invited to lunch at Keynsham House where he noted, with admiration (but perhaps a little prosaically), 'the business-like way in which [she] carved the sirloin of beef'.[4] Later, he became impressed by her acting ability after she gave a memorable performance as Dot, the inquisitive maid-servant in the popular farce, *Ticklish Times*, as part of the Whishaws' private theatricals party.

When ETW's attention was not fixed on Mary, it was now directed at making a contribution to Cheltenham's local community. In January 1861 he became Secretary of the Working Men's Club. There, he lectured on various subjects, the first being one which was to prove a lifelong professional interest: 'Health and how to preserve it'. In a different field, he contributed to the newly-formed local Working Naturalists' Association, whose fifteen members' aim was 'the systematic examination and collection of flora and fauna within ten miles of Cheltenham'.[5] Sharing out the responsibility of compiling authenticated lists of plants, animals and fossils, they divided up the tasks based on members' personal interests and expertise. ETW and his friend Dr Abercrombie were given responsibility for diatomaceae and desmids (both types of microscopic green algae that occur in freshwater). Fascinated by these minute organisms the two friends collected what ETW considered a 'very incomplete' list of eighty-seven species.[6] It was a subject he would return to in later life.[7]

By the summer of 1862, ETW's passion for Mary was unabated. He seized every opportunity to spend time in her company. When considering which church to attend, he chose St John's: partly attracted by its preacher, he also knew that Mary was already a regular attender. After the services, the two lovers would exchange admiring glances and swap social pleasantries. Nevertheless, conventions of the day prevented them from spending time alone together. Any walks, boating trips or rides they were able to arrange together had to be chaperoned, usually by one of Mary's brothers. Frustrated by the lack of opportunity to pour out his innermost feelings, on 12 July ETW decided to propose to Mary by letter. He waited anxiously for the reply but when, finally, the response came, he was hugely disappointed - so much so that he decided to let off steam by running the 7 miles to Gloucester, only returning to Cheltenham on the midnight train.

Two days later, he returned to Hean Castle to welcome Charly back from British Columbia after four years' work for the North American

Boundary Commission to demarcate the boundary between the Canadian colonies and the United States. Charly had traversed swamps, prairies, primeval forests and mountain peaks, and had a fund of tales to tell. He had survived some of the hardest winters on record, and met plenty of rattlesnakes.[8] All these stories gave ETW some welcome distraction from his rejected proposal.

There were other engagements and distractions too: a trip to London to visit the Crystal Palace and see Auber's opera *Masaniello*; a demonstration by an electro-biologist (this confirmed ETW's belief in the medical value of hypnotism); his establishment, in May 1863, of Cheltenham's first medical library;[9] and the thrill of seeing his brother Rathmel victorious at Cheltenham College sports day. Rathmel not only won the walking race after beating Frederick Carrington (1844-1913), later Major General Sir Frederick Carrington,[10] but also gained the heavyweight boxing belt which had been offered up by Carrington. There was also a meeting with Dr William Lawrence (1783-1867), a leading surgeon at St Bartholomew's hospital. Apart from excelling as a medical professional Dr Lawrence also achieved recognition for two books he published early in his career, which outlined pre-Darwinian ideas on evolution and man's nature, a topic which interested ETW greatly. Impressed by his 'noble carriage and dignified manner' and describing him as 'a man among men', ETW recalled:

> It was during [Dr Lawrence's] last illness, suffering from Aphasia (loss of speech) the medical men were in doubt, when he asked for pen and ink with which he made blot after blot on the paper – what his meaning could be when it occurred to one of them that 'Black Drop' an obsolete preparation of opium was meant – and on mentioning it the patient at once became calm and content.[11]

Meanwhile, at Hean Castle the storm that had been threatening on the horizon for the past few years suddenly broke: the entire estate had to be sold. 'We knew not how nor why – indeed the mystery has never been cleared', wrote ETW.[12] Under his father's ownership the estate had been significantly improved: he had encouraged good husbandry and cleared land to make it more productive; but he had also been too indulgent with rents and had lost significant sums of money in the production of

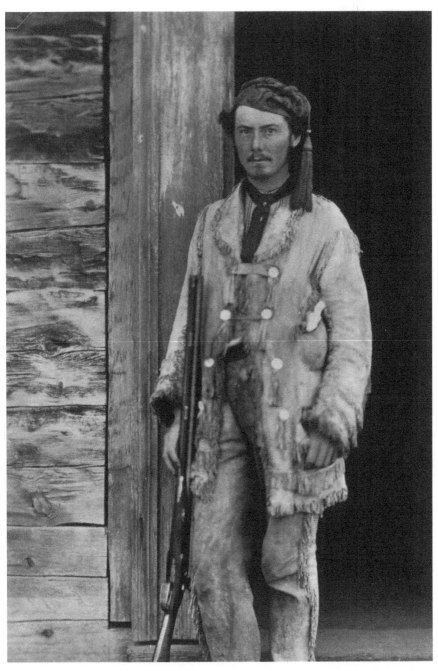

Lieutenant Charles Wilson, R.E., Secretary of the North American Boundary Commission.

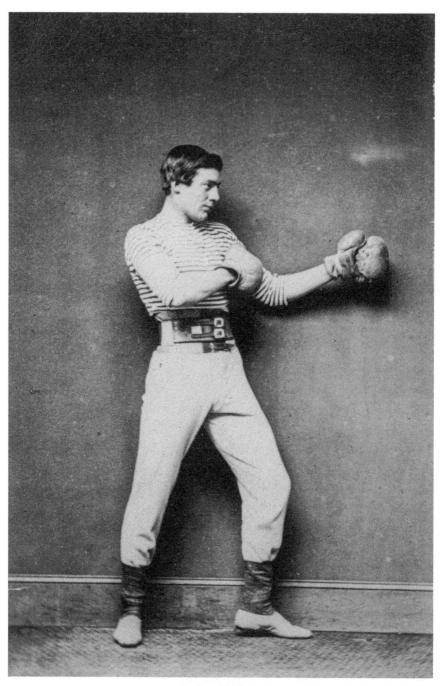

Rathmel Wilson.

firebricks and iron. The estate went under the hammer in Tenby on 9 September 1863 and was sold for £30,000, a sum that took into account that the 'anthracite coal found under the estate commanded in London as high a price as any found in the kingdom'.[13] Although ETW was by now earning a living, he still partly depended on additional income from home, and the loss of Hean Castle caused him some anxiety.

After returning to Cheltenham in January 1864, ETW's disappointments were soon replaced by feelings of hope. At a ball given by Countess Stenbock, née Lucy Sophia Frerichs (1840-96),[14] the daughter of a Manchester cotton industrialist, he was surprised and delighted to see Mary again, despite her parents expressly forbidding her to maintain any contact with him. They happily spent the evening together, rekindling their friendship. Around this time, other friendships - with the staff at Cheltenham College - were also being strengthened. ETW was delighted when he was given the freedom of the College and treated in every respect as if he were an Old Cheltonian.

By the summer, the full impact of losing Hean Castle was brought home when ETW's parents and sisters arrived in Cheltenham to take lodgings at 12 Spa Buildings[15] overlooking Montpellier Gardens. ETW left his own lodgings and made the short journey across the gardens to join his family. While Mary was constantly in his thoughts, his professional attention was now focused on preparing an important paper on Cheltenham's sanitary statistics.

The production of reliable, accurate sanitary statistics as an indicator of the health of a place had concerned him for some time. The subject already had a long and chequered history. By the 1830s, life tables for various towns and cities were already in existence, but these were unsatisfactory and often contradictory. Liverpool, ETW's birthplace, for instance, was considered one of the healthiest places in England, the increase in its population being attributed to factors such as the salubrity of its air.[16] The claim was backed up by deductions based on simple burial returns. However, once General Registration of births, marriages and deaths was introduced in 1837, the sanitary state of the country could be established on a much more systematic statistical basis. Even the first returns were revealing, indicating, for instance, that overcrowding and density of population went hand in hand with increased mortality rates. Such was the optimism following the publication of the Registrar-

General's first report that some believed doctors would one day learn to 'administer remedies with discrimination, and with due reference to the circumstances of the population' based on their understanding of 'the extent to which epidemics vary in different locations, seasons, and classes of society'.[17]

While ETW shared this utopian vision, he also recognised that – nearly three decades later - its practical realisation was still fraught with difficulties. It was something, he thought, that could be well illustrated through presenting a case study of a town like Cheltenham. Receiving encouragement from trusted medical friends, he took the plunge and presented his paper[18] at the Bath meeting of the British Association for the Advancement of Science on 16 September 1864. The paper was well received in both the professional and local press. Today, it can be recognised as a pioneering epidemiological study, which illustrated how attempts to gain a wholly accurate picture of a town's sanitation were complicated by various factors. In Cheltenham's case, these included responsibility for sewers being divided between the local authority and private undertakings; the differing sources and supplies of drinking water; and the diverse make-up and mobility of the town's population which made it difficult to precisely identify and balance the various factors affecting the likelihood of disease and death. ETW also drew attention to the increase in pauperism in the town, which was well above the national average, and the fact that Cheltenham's death-rate statistics had been distorted by the inclusion of figures from its wider agricultural district. One reviewer commented:

> Dr. Wilson, in an admirable Essay on Cheltenham, proved with the sternness of Roman Justice that the town proper, the sub-district, cannot yet claim a lower average death-rate than 19 per 1,000, and that its mortality is somewhat above that of the wide agricultural district on which it stands.[19]

Buoyed up with this success and keen to pursue his sanitary utopia, ETW proceeded with a more detailed study of the town, mindful of the various imperfections of the new system of registration: inclusion of a cause of death was not yet compulsory; and discrepancies could arise between those deaths which were certified and those which were not. Added to this were cases of fraud or carelessness in certifying and recording deaths accurately; conscious decisions made to disguise the truth, for instance in deaths from cancer and syphilis; and frequent uncertainties about the primary cause when two or more diseases were involved. There could also be simple clerical errors, or mistakes made when records were aggregated into quarterly and annual reports.

Another major shortcoming in the system, ETW felt, was 'the fact that registration of death and registration of disease [were being] used indifferently to describe the certified entry of the cause of death'.[20] In an 1869 article for the *British and Foreign Medico-chirurgical Review*, he set out a detailed case to show that 'the cause of death [was] no safe indication of the prevalence or fatality of disease, and that the conversion of a mortuary record into a health barometer [was] to the last degree mischievous and the results untrue'.[21] He argued:

> It would be well, therefore, if local effort could be made in some sense to supplement the shortcomings of the national returns – if local knowledge of topography, meteorology, drainage, water supply, social conditions and all those circumstances which more immediately affect a people's well-being, could be brought to bear upon the interpretation of local records of sickness and disease.[22]

This was now something he set out to achieve.

3
Pioneering Photography (1865)

Cheltenham Photographic Society – Photomicrography –
Photozincography

*'We were there working together on all spare evenings at Photomicrography
and very engrossing it was, though from want of proper appliances and having
to use artificial light it took a great deal of time'.*
~ ETW ~

A T THE BEGINNING OF 1865, ETW's interest in photography, first
ignited in student days through his family connection with Francis
Frith, entered a significant new phase. To quote his words directly: 'The
year 1865 was a memorable one to me. I got back to Cheltenham on

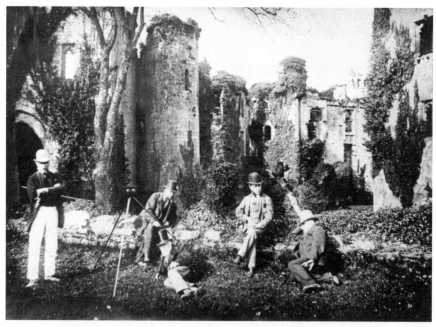

A Cheltenham Photographic Society outing to Raglan Castle, 1875.

January 3 and next day the first Photographic Society was started with Dr. Abercrombie as President while I acted as Secretary'.[1] Thus began Cheltenham's Photographic Society, the sixth earliest in the country, and still flourishing today.[2]

Although photography as a technology and a pursuit had been steadily growing throughout the first half of the nineteenth century, it was London's Great Exhibition of 1851 which marked a real turning point. When ETW visited it at the age of eighteen he probably witnessed (amongst the other exhibits of machines, tools and appliances from all around the world) the world's first major exhibition of photography. Here, inside the Crystal Palace at Hyde Park, one could see the latest achievements of photographers from America, France and Great Britain. From then on, photography would receive official recognition and start to take shape as a serious movement.[3]

Six months before he and Abercrombie launched the Cheltenham Photographic Society, ETW had recognised the important influence that photography was now making 'on our habits, our tastes, and social institutions'. He marvelled at how photography, 'the wonder of yesterday', had now become 'the social necessity of to-day', contributing so much to our comfort, luxuries and requirements.[4] Although he appreciated how privileged he was to be able to rub shoulders with those who could still remember the first cameras 'and the mysterious powers with which their imagination invested it', he was equally fascinated by the earliest origins of the technology which, he considered, were 'involved in as much mystery as that of any of the arts ... [deriving] from the earliest ages of civilization'.[5] As an example, he referred to research at the time which indicated the possibility of 'sun pictures' being taken by James Watt and Matthew Boulton as early as 1792 but, because their techniques were apparently lost or unrecorded, a new starting point had to be found in the experiments of Wedgwood and Sir Humphrey Davy in 1802.

By the time ETW first visited Cheltenham in 1853, professional photographers had already been long established along the town's Promenade. Following the invention of the daguerreotype process by Louis-Jacques-Mandé Daguerre in 1839, which for the first time allowed photographic portraits to be made, commercial studios started to appear up and down the country. Fashionable Cheltenham was one of the first towns to open a studio[6] when a certain John Palmer set up his business in

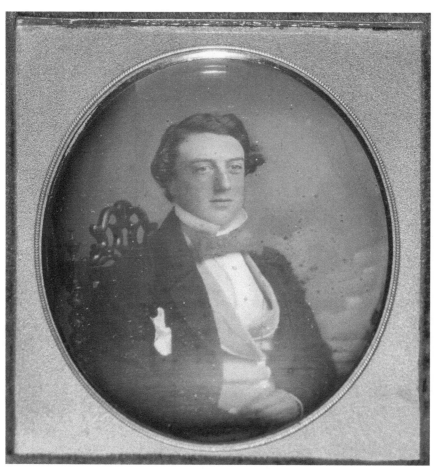

A hand-coloured daguerreotype of ETW, by Richard Lowe.

September 1841.[7] Another early practitioner was Richard Lowe (b. c.1823), who arrived in Cheltenham from his native America in 1850. After opening the Cheltenham Photographic Institution (located on the Promenade) in June, he advertised 'his new method of taking Photographic Pictures by the aid of *electricity* … to obtain the most beautiful Daguerreotype Portraits, in the darkest rainy weather in from 10 to 20 seconds'.[8] It was probably in 1853 that ETW visited Lowe's studio to have his own portrait taken. The quality of Lowe's work is evident from this image, and one can readily imagine the interesting conversation that the photographer and his subject might have had on the technical aspects of the process.[9] Any further contact between the two would have been abruptly curtailed when in 1856, to general surprise, the American left town in a great hurry to return home, sailing across the Atlantic from Liverpool. He left behind a string of debts, having bought a £35 gold watch, £40 of plate, and £22 of drapery.[10]

At first, the cost of studio photographs was high everywhere, typically a guinea per portrait, including a frame or morocco case.[11] Yet the demand for cheaper portraits and *cartes de visite* soon meant that they became more affordable; and by 1865, there were as many as seventeen photographers working in Cheltenham alone.[12] Popular as portraiture remained, it was only part of the demand. Within two years, John Palmer's business was taking photographic commissions for houses, buildings and works of fine art.[13]

ETW's earliest experience of photography dated from 1854 when he used the wet-collodion process to develop glass plates. While the process produced satisfactory levels of detail and clarity in the resulting images, it also necessitated speed given that immediate developing and fixing was required before the collodion film had time to dry. On one occasion he remembered photographing a subject some distance from his dark room, but to achieve success he had to set up his camera beforehand 'and then gallop the distance to and fro on a fast pony'.[14] Another drawback was that his hands were almost permanently stained with the colour of mahogany through usage of the chemicals.

By the beginning of 1865, ETW had acquired much valuable practical knowledge and experience of photography, both for portraiture and for recording social and geographical landscapes. As early as 1855, he had struck up a close friendship with the prolific travelling photographer Francis Frith, whom he knew through his Aunt Susan. Frith was one of the great pioneers of his day, experimenting with the use of glass negatives and earning the reputation of being able to 'carry us far beyond anything that is in the power of the most accomplished artist to transfer to his canvas'.[15] Frith not only embarked upon a colossal project to photograph every town and village in the UK but also gained widespread fame for travelling to Africa, even venturing beyond the sixth cataract of the Nile. Once, ETW had to stand in the foreground for twenty minutes while Frith took a picture. He recalled:

His [Frith's] first real effort was with a sort of van adapted to the purpose and fitted up as a dark room - with this he travelled through North Wales,

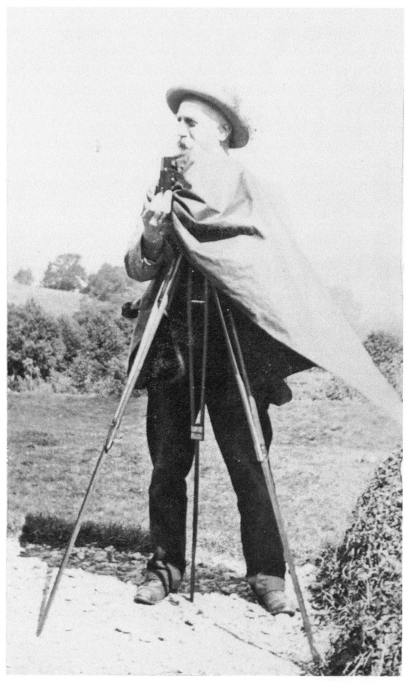

ETW with tripod, c.1892.

and the sale of his pictures not only covered all expenses but brought in a handsome profit as well. This encouraged him to make the still more arduous but more profitable venture in Egypt.[16]

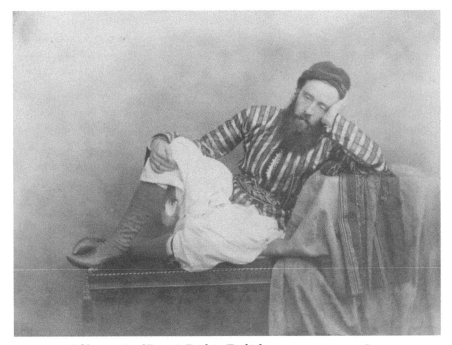

Self-portrait of Francis Frith in Turkish summer costume, 1857.

On another occasion, ETW and Frith, the latter having recently returned from another tour in North Wales, drove a brougham with yellow blinds all through London to Winchmore Hill. This spectacle attracted much attention and caused considerable amusement to passers-by: as ETW noted, 'it resembled a van for a dwarf or other show'.[17]

While ETW enjoyed landscape and portrait photography throughout his life, as a scientist his heart lay in photography's potential as a tool for recording 'an absolute knowledge of the visible world'.[18] It was through his friendship with Dr Abercrombie that his passion for photography began to coalesce with science. As well as their shared background in medicine and sports, central to their friendship was their interest in photography. In particular, ETW recalled many pleasant 'evenings by lamplight' which he spent with Dr Abercrombie engaged in photomicrography.

Photomicrography is the process by which a photograph is taken through a microscope to show a magnified image of an object, not to be confused with microphotography (where a microscope is used to view highly miniaturised photographs). ETW considered microphotography images as frivolous curiosities of the time, typically showing minute portraits or views, but later the serious uses of the technique began to be recognised during the Franco-Prussian war in 1870 when microphotography was first used to transfer sensitive information.

Although many pioneers were involved in the early development of photomicrography, it was the Revd Joseph B. Reade (1801-70) who astounded the scientific world when he exhibited the magnified image of a flea at a soirée given by the Marquis of Northampton, President of the Royal Society, on 27 April 1839.[19] Before then, science had relied on the fidelity of human eye and hand to capture and record objects seen through the microscopic lens. Now, this new branch of photography promised to present reality unfiltered by 'the unconscious impress of [the artist's] mind'.[20] Moreover, it would present the microscopic world at first hand, objectively, in all its glory, and do so easily, accurately and cheaply. More importantly, ETW believed, photomicrography could resolve all questions of scientific doubt: through permanently fixing with unerring accuracy the minutest differences, changes in growth and development could be recorded for study and comparisons made over time.[21]

Influenced by Dr Richard Maddox (1816-1902)[22] and other leading photomicrography experts of the day, ETW himself made important advances in the use of artificial light for photomicrography. Aware of the benefits of being able to achieve consistent results, independent of seasonal variations and dark days, he identified easier and cheaper approaches. Apart from making the complex techniques more accessible and affordable to the ordinary practitioner, he also promoted the art of photomicrography as a pleasurable and inspiring activity that should be enjoyed. He wrote:

In the uninterrupted quiet of a long winter's evening, by a comfortable fire, the student of natural phenomena has everything at his command, and is enabled to record with a faithfulness otherwise unattainable many interesting appearances which would otherwise be irretrievably lost.[23]

The method, which ETW and Abercrombie used (see Appendix 2), was originally published in the *Popular Science Review*, and later summarised in Lionel Beale's *How to work with the microscope*.[24] The calibration of their equipment, necessary because they needed set magnifications to support a scientific study, involved a large number of exposures. Each exposure involved plate preparation, exposure and development for each objective lens and magnification. This required dogged persistence. When working with an oil lamp, for example, they had to make

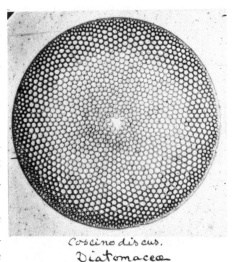

Coscino discus.
Diatomaceæ

Groups of Diatomaceae, an example of ETW's photomicrography.

30-minute exposures. This would be appropriately adjusted when using lime light, magnesium flash, or daylight. The printed results they achieved were described as 'remarkably good', possessing 'a peculiar delicacy in the half-tones and shadows, with much roundness of the objects'.[25] One reviewer commented:

> All of the general characteristic appearances of the objects are exceedingly perfect and the simplicity of the apparatus, and the immense advantage of the efficient illumination in all weathers, are great advantages.[26]

However, it was not just photomicrography which fascinated ETW. There were other innovative photographic techniques that also attracted his attention. One of these was photozincography,[27] which was invented in 1859 under the leadership of Colonel Sir Henry James (1803-77), the Director-General of the Ordnance Survey in Southampton. ETW first met James when visiting Charly who had recently taken up an appointment in the Topographical Department. This method of printing an image from a zinc plate after it had been prepared through a photo-lithographic process attracted ETW's interest because of its ability to provide accurate

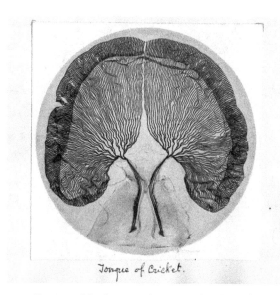

Tongue of Cricket.

Tongue of Cricket, another example of ETW's photomicrography.

and finely detailed copies of photographs. James showed ETW interesting examples of what photozincographs could achieve, including reproductions of ancient maps and documents which ETW was able to compare with the originals; among these were manuscript letters of Queen Elizabeth I and Mary, Queen of Scots. For ETW, photozincography presented a potential solution to one of early photography's biggest concerns, that of permanency. He wrote:

> We are working for the day only, without a thought for the future. "Things of beauty", which should be "joys for ever," will be fading away when we have learned to value them most; the treasures of a generation will pass slowly and irrevocably from our possession.[28]

Therefore, he welcomed the attempts to substitute carbon compounds for silver to help with permanency, but also recognised the potential of photozincography to make it easier to reproduce good quality images on a very large scale through transferring the negative for printing from glass to etched zinc. After being inspired by James, ETW was keen to put theory into practice. For several long evenings, he experimented with Dr Abercrombie on photozincography, and then shared his knowledge through a paper presented to the Cheltenham Photographic Society. For ETW, photography was to remain a lifelong passion, and it was also to play an important part in his next big project.

4
The Quest for Clean Drinking Water (1865)

Cheltenham's water supply controversy – Evidence to Houses of
Parliament – 'Water in its relation to health'

*'... a people's health is undermined by the consumption of such minute
quantities of a subtle poison as may be contained in their daily water supply'.*
~ ETW ~

JUST ONE MONTH AFTER launching Cheltenham's Photographic
Society, ETW threw himself into the vortex of a debate concerning the
town's water supply. The story of how Cheltenham came to obtain a reliable
supply of clean drinking water is long, complicated and characterised by a
remarkable amount of angry debate and political controversy.[1] Originally,
the town had relied on private wells and rainwater tanks before a private
company was formed in 1824 to provide piped water for those willing to
pay. This led to the creation of three classes of consumers:

> ... those who could pay for mains water: those who obtained their water
> free from private wells and those, notably the poor, who obtained their
> water where they could, either from a limited number of public pumps,
> streams or from a water carrier who sold [it] from a cart.[2]

However, there were 'frequent complaints that the Water Company
provided an inadequate and intermittent supply'.[3] By 1865, the situation
had reached a particular crisis-point. Apart from increasing demands from
a recent growth in population, there were concerns about a deterioration
in the overall quality of the water supply. Something needed to be done,
and two possible solutions were put forward. The first suggested exploiting
the Boxwell springs from South Cerney. This was immediately rejected by
the Oxford authorities who were alarmed at the thought of diverting the
springs away from the River Thames into the Severn, since it would have
involved abstracting approximately one million gallons of water per day.
The alternative scheme, which was proposed by the Waterworks Company,

involved obtaining the water from the River Severn itself. In view of the
fact that Cheltenham's supply could not be obtained from the watershed
in the local district, and the town could not trespass on neighbouring
supplies, The *Cheltenham Looker-On* urged its readers to support the
Severn scheme based on the following logic:

> ... though the water thence procured may not, in the first instance, be quite
> so pure as that of the mountain rivulets which had formerly sufficed for
> the necessities of the Town, it is, unquestionably, better than that with
> which the inhabitants have been recently supplied from the sandbed;
> and, at all events, cannot be inferior to that which the Metropolis receives
> from the Thames, and upon which a population exceeding two millions are
> wholly dependent.[4]

ETW disagreed vehemently and immediately wrote a letter to the
more Liberal-leaning *Cheltenham Examiner*[5] questioning the desirability
of obtaining drinking water from the River Severn and stressing the
importance of making the right decision lest Cheltenham's title as the
'Queen of Watering Places' be put at risk and epidemics break out from
water-borne diseases such as cholera and typhoid. He wrote:

> Can anything be more unwise? Can anything be more hazardous? Can
> anything be more opposed to all the laborious teachings of sanitary
> science, than to draw a supply of drinking water for a large and important
> town from a sewage-tainted source?[6]

ETW identified two additional options which, he felt, should be
brought into the equation: the possibility of obtaining the supply from the
Cotswolds, or, as a last resort, continuing with the *status quo*. In essence,
ETW considered, it was really a choice between water from a sewage-laden
tidal river and the pure source of water from the local hills. When it came to
considering the former, he pointed to irrefutable evidence why this option
should be rejected. Firstly, there were two independent scientific studies
which strongly advised against the River Severn on grounds of its poor
water quality. In addition, there were significant amounts of sewage that
flowed directly into the river from an aggregate population of one million
people; there was constant drainage and run-off from 6,000 square miles

of intensively manured land adjacent to the river; and there were frequent sightings of dead carcasses and insect pupal cases, as well as waste dumped from barges and steamers. On the other hand, there were good indications of a plentiful, clean and reliable supply from the Cotswolds which could be augmented through borings made to tap into the water-bearing strata on the eastern side.

The question of whether the River Severn was to be used as a supply of drinking water, in the interim at least, was to be finally settled in Parliament. The Water Company raised a Bill which was initially debated before a House of Commons committee on 21 March. ETW was asked to give evidence along with Dr Thomas Wright (1809-84), a fellow physician at Cheltenham General Hospital and Dispensary; they appeared as expert witnesses, speaking on behalf of the Town Commissioners who were in opposition to the Bill. ETW recorded that the 'wrangling of opposing Engineers and doctors was highly entertaining' and, memorably, Dr Wright remarked at the hearing that a drinking supply should, like Caesar's wife, be 'above suspicion'.[7] ETW supplied photographs as part of his evidence to demonstrate the existence of fungus caused by sewage contamination in the tanks of Severn water at Worcester. Despite their efforts, the Bill was not rejected, so a further appeal was made to the House of Lords.

Before this hearing took place, further debate in Cheltenham reached fever pitch: between April and May three protest meetings were held against the Severn scheme. ETW was again in the thick of action. He followed up his concerns about the dangers of making the wrong decision by giving a lecture at the Working Men's Club. Choosing as his title 'Water in its relation to health',[8] he sought to dispel some common myths and to give simple, clear scientific facts so that the local inhabitants would be better informed. He highlighted the following guidelines:

Drinking water should be: 1, without smell of any kind; 2, without any special taste; 3, transparent and colourless, without any deposit; 4, cool and well aerated, like soda water; 5, containing a moderate amount of solid matter, and of an innocent character; 6, a certain proportion only of the solid matter should be organic, and never animal.[9]

As a cautionary tale, he quoted the case of a well in Broad Street, London, previously celebrated for its good quality water: more than

500 people had died within a week from an outbreak of cholera after it was contaminated with sewage. This was the case which the physician John Snow (1813-58), later widely recognised as 'the father of modern epidemiology', used to prove that cholera was spread by water and not airborne miasma, as previously thought. ETW's intent was not to scaremonger but to present his arguments with clear scientific evidence. Recognising the difficulty of proving a connection between cause and effect when such minute quantities of a subtle poison are involved, he urged his audience to drink only the purest water and to carry out their own qualitative tests. These included guarding 'against a water which became offensive on being warmed, a water that would not keep in a transparent and colourless state, or that left a brownish or white deposit in the cisterns'.[10] He thought these were likely to be more infallible than other tests, even those carried out by chemists who, in ETW's experience, sometimes failed to distinguish between harmless algae and noxious fungal growths.

When it came to the Severn question, his message was clear: while the river water was suitable for the purposes of washing, this was not the case for drinking. 'The Severn,' he commented, 'may, probably before long, be cleansed of its greatest impurities by legislative enactment; but even then, it could not vie with the supply from the hill slopes'.[11]

In June, ETW and Dr Wright returned to the Houses of Parliament, armed with further photographic evidence showing fungal growth in the Severn water tanks at Worcester.[12] This time, the Bill was successfully defeated. Nevertheless, an adequate long-term solution had still not been achieved. It was a subject to which ETW would repeatedly return.

5
Friendship and Marriage (1865-67)

Bachelors' Ball – Reacquaintance with the Whishaws – Marriage –
Honeymoon in France and Italy – Birth of Lilian – Friends in Council

*'... I was greeted by a friendly smile from the top of a brake, which seemed to
encourage a renewal of acquaintance though upon what terms was a question
still to be solved.'*
~ ETW ~

WHILE PHOTOMICROGRAPHY AND THE quest for a supply of clean
drinking water occupied much of ETW's mind in 1865, there was
still time for relaxation and social engagement. During February, he
went to numerous parties, including one hosted by Lieutenant Colonel
William Nicol Burns, the son of the poet Robert Burns, where he enjoyed
a clandestine chat with Mary; and then there was the Bachelors' Ball, one
of the most significant events in Cheltenham's social calendar, which he
helped to sponsor. Taking place on 27 February, at the Assembly Rooms[1]
on Cheltenham's High Street, the ball, organised for fancy dress, was
a way 'of reciprocating the hospitalities [the bachelors had] received
from their friends during the Season'.[2] Among the 350 guests was ETW
dressed in Greek costume, a choice possibly inspired by a desire to dress
in harmony with the town's Grecian architecture.[3] As the crowds made
their way through the vestibule, richly decorated with flowers, flags, and
silken banners, they entered the ballroom where they were enthralled by
'a circular mirror, around which a number of swords were arranged, so as
to form a species of wheel, the blades glistening brightly in the gas-light'.[4]
The Grecian-looking figure mingled freely, conversing with a baffling
number of characters:

Here an Indian chieftain, conspicuous for the richness of his savage
dress, might be seen in friendly converse with Mary Queen of Scots or
her maidens, or on chatting terms with bluff King Hal, who was by no
means the least noticeable of the many noteworthy characters. In another

part, Mephistopheles might be seen in close proximity to a Puritan lady, or a Syrian belle, or talking unconcernedly to a Franciscan monk. A barrister full robed and wigged was thinking of anything but his briefs; and courtiers, nymphs, a Knight Templar, and Nights and Mornings, were mingled together in inextricable confusion.

Apart from dancing several well-known valses, galops, lancers, waltzes and mazurkas, the assembled company also enjoyed several quadrilles. A sumptuous banquet was served at around one o'clock in the morning, after which dancing was resumed. It was not until half-past five in the morning that the last quadrille was danced and the ball 'of almost unexampled brilliancy' finally came to an end.

Another opportunity for relaxation occurred during the summer of 1865 when ETW visited Cornwall with his friend Charles Cave, who dabbled in art. Apart from bathing they devoted themselves to creative pursuits, Cave's sketchpad and ETW's camera trying to capture the subtlety and magnificence of the coastline between Fowey, the Lizard Peninsula and Penzance. On their way back, they stayed in Ilfracombe where ETW's family had once settled for a time. Here, ETW's heart suddenly began to beat faster after being amazed to discover that the Whishaws had also chosen Ilfracombe as their holiday destination. Soon he was 'greeted by a friendly smile from the top of a brake',[5] Mary clearly signalling her desire to renew their friendship.

At first, ETW was uncertain about the terms upon which Mary's parents would allow him to renew his acquaintance with their daughter, but by September they were being allowed to have private conversations together. After evening service at church one day, they strolled up Capstone Hill, enjoying the breath-taking views along the North Devon coast, when ETW plucked up courage to, once again, propose to Mary. This time, the answer was favourable, Mary immediately accepting without hesitation. The couple's 'psychological moment'[6] had finally arrived. They excitedly made their way down the hill in the gloaming light and conveyed the news to Mary's parents. Once again, however, to their great disappointment Mary's mother reacted negatively. The following day, she forbade any communication between the happy couple. Despite this, at the beginning of October, ETW suddenly received one of the most important telegrams in his life - a message from his beloved, reporting that 'all is as we wish'.[7]

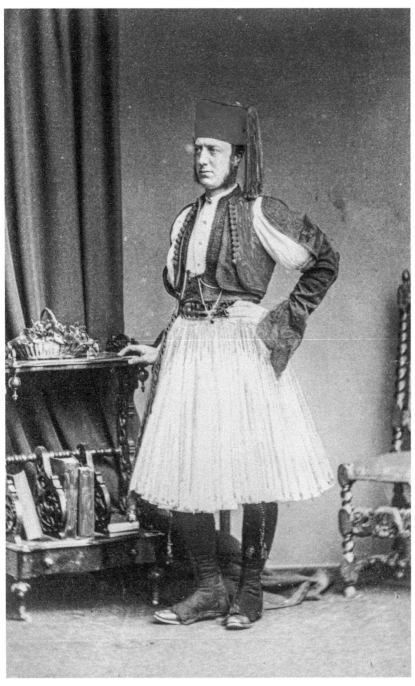

ETW in Greek costume.

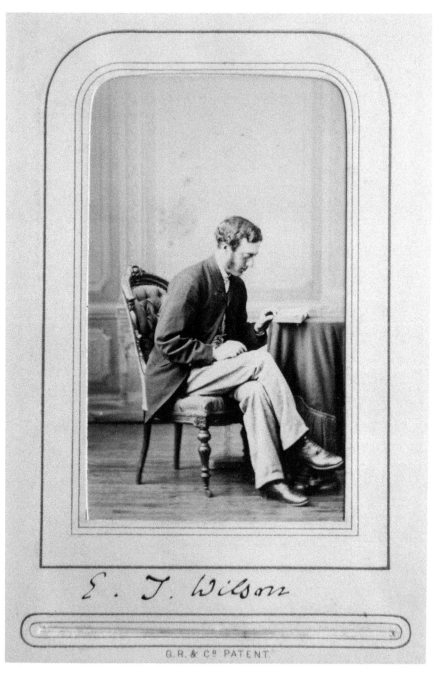

Portrait of ETW, from the Friends in Council Archive.

By the evening, he was being welcomed with open arms and, in the days that followed, they resumed their courtship, interspersing long walks and rides with visits to see relatives at Great Rollright and trips to local churches to make brass rubbings.

Later that year, in Cheltenham, ETW moved a short distance from his lodgings in Montpellier Terrace to number 6 (now 91), which his father had purchased for him and his brother Harry. The following year, excitement grew as ETW and Mary made preparations for their wedding day; further excitement arose on 24 March when ETW fulfilled a lifetime's wish to attend a performance of readings by Charles Dickens, renowned for his perfect elocution and excellent power of mimicry. The Assembly Rooms were packed as he witnessed the exceptional performance by 'Boz' who brought various scenes from his novels to life, including the trial scene from *Pickwick Papers* and the death of Little Nell. ETW vividly recalled the novelist 'with his sparkling black eyes and mobile face throwing himself wholly into the reading and making one take part in the scene'.[8]

Less than a month following this red-letter day, ETW and Mary were finally able to enjoy their 'day of days'[9] when they got married on 18 April 1866 at St Luke's Church, Cheltenham. Relatives and friends packed the Early English style church, built in 1853-4 partly to cater for pupils of nearby Cheltenham College and the fashionable Sandford district where many of their families resided.[10] Following the service, the guests adjourned to the reception held at Linden House,[11] the Whishaws' new family home. It was such a significant event in the town's social calendar that the *Cheltenham Chronicle* commented that it conferred 'upon that particular week of the season quite a distinctive character'.[12] The notable absentee was Charly who, at that time, was undertaking a ground-breaking survey of Palestine. Their honeymoon brought the delights of Paris, Avignon and Marseilles, from whence they continued their journey along the Riviera to Genoa, Milan and the Italian Lakes, returning via tunnels cut through the avalanches that still lingered in the French Alps.

Just over a year after their marriage, on 27 May 1867, Mary gave birth to their first child, Lilian Mary (see Appendix 1 for ETW's family tree). Around this time, ETW was also elected to a small club 'established for purposes of Intellectual Entertainment' known as Friends in Council (FiC).[13]

Friends in Council Attendance Card 1895-6.

Founded at the home of Major Robert Cary Barnard (1827-1906)[14] on 14 October 1862, the society derived its name from the volumes of discourses on social issues conveyed as conversations among a group of friends by Sir Arthur Helps.[15] Regarded as possibly 'the oldest Literary Society in the West of England',[16] the FiC (now comprising fifteen members) was then limited to twelve, following the recommendation from one of its other founding members, Henry Alfred James,[17] the Vice-Principal of St Paul's College, who had belonged to the Cambridge Apostles when a student at Trinity College. Today, the FiC still meets monthly in members' houses, the host being appointed President for the evening. The atmosphere engendered at the meetings appealed strongly to ETW and, during 1912, when the society celebrated its jubilee year, he was acknowledged as its most senior surviving member. A review of the papers read by ETW during a period spanning forty-two years reveals a remarkable breadth of interests, covering a wealth of literary, scientific and socio-political subjects.[18]

While the talks were invariably interesting and informative, and explicitly excluded coverage of current political and theological topics, ETW amusingly recalled one curious evening in October 1870 when John Walker, a recently elected new member who was also a member of the Council of Cheltenham College, proposed the subject of billiards for his talk. Given that Walker was a Cambridge mathematician, the members expected 'a learned inquisition on the dynamics of the game'.[19] ETW continued:

> ... after a few preliminary remarks by our host on the Social advantages of a Billiard table in the house, we were invited to a practical application of the game as being preferable to a paper - and in a very short time the most ancient and staid of the Friends might have been seen renewing their youth in their shirt sleeves and with cues in their hands making cannons and losing hazards - Though very generous and hospitable John Walker soon found himself out of his element in a literary society and his resignation followed soon after.[20]

The society introduced him to some of the greatest local intellects of the day, including the Revd Henry Hayman (1823-1904),[21] Headmaster of Cheltenham Grammar School from 1859 to 1868, the Revd T. W. Norwood, an expert in geology, and the Revd George Butler (1819-90), who was vice principal at Cheltenham College. Perhaps the most famous was the celebrated Shakespearean actor William Charles Macready (1793-1873), a close friend of Charles Dickens, who was elected to the FiC one year earlier than ETW, having come to retire at 6 Wellington Square in Pittville. Both ETW and another member, the physician Dr Claudius Buchanan Ker (1821-98), a friend of Alfred Tennyson, fondly recalled lectures given by Macready on Shakespeare. Conveying the inherent quality of these meetings, Ker recalled 'the extreme modesty with which [Macready] gave his opinions on a subject in which he was a master, while every face was turned towards him'.[22] 'His words were worthy of all our attention', he continued, '- measured, beautifully chosen, and representing the very essence of true criticism'.[23] The FiC also helped ETW to forge closer relationships with those friends he knew from other circles. They included John Middleton, already established as a church architect, the Revd Joseph Fenn, vicar of Christ Church, and the Revds Alfred Barry, William Dobson and Herbert Kynaston, who served as Principals of Cheltenham College. Apart from providing ETW with valuable friendships and intellectual stimulation it also provided opportunities for other members of ETW's family to enjoy FiC meetings when he hosted meetings at home.

6
District Nursing (1867-70)

The Cheltenham Nursing Institution – Inquest into death of a flyman
– Insufficient water supply – Births of Bernard and Nellie – Palestine
Exploration Fund – Advancement through the medical profession

The nurses of old were odious creatures
'Gamp' their name and coarse their features
With their bottle and 'brolly' they took possession
And laughed in the face of the old profession
But we've changed all that, and the Nurse of today
Would look on the Gamps with grim dismay ... .[1]
~ ETW ~

DESPITE THE HEFTY PRICE of tickets to hear Charles Dickens perform three readings at Cheltenham's Assembly Rooms on 22 January 1869, the packed audience reserved their heartiest applause for the novelist's final reading of the evening, his rendition of 'the oddities and comicalities of Mrs Gamp'.[2] Dickens' celebrated portrayal of Sarah Gamp[3] is one of an incompetent gin-swilling domiciliary nurse and midwife who cares more about her own welfare than that of her patients. Gamp was used by many Victorian medical reformers as a symbol of all that was perceived as reprehensible in old-style nursing, in contrast to the committed, professional, and morally-upright figure of Florence Nightingale, widely recognised as the founder of modern nursing.

Ten years earlier, William Rathbone (1819-1902), a Liverpool merchant and philanthropist, established a nursing school in the city. This supplied trained nurses for its eighteen districts, from which organised 'district nursing' evolved as an important part of health care provision. Thereafter, a number of provincial schemes also came about, including one initiated by ETW in Cheltenham. 'In October 1867 at my suggestion', he wrote, 'a nurse's home was quietly started in the Christ Church district ...'.[4] Prior to this, hospital-trained nurses were practically unheard of in the town, unless they were temporarily imported from London, Bristol, or Gloucester. Later known as the Cheltenham Nursing Institution, the organisation (located at 6 Lansdown Parade, with a Lady Superintendent next door at No.5) was run by Canon J. F. Fenn, the vicar of Christ Church and a member of Friends in Council, and funded by the congregation. ETW acted as secretary, specified the rules, and arranged for the nurses to be trained in the Gloucestershire Infirmary. Initially employing a single nurse dedicated to serving the sick poor of Christ Church district, and a small number of supplementary nurses available for private families, by 1870 the staff comprised eight nurses for private families, and one for district work. Significantly, the nurses generated glowing testimonials for their efficiency and kindness which provided 'a gratifying proof that the institution [was] doing good work, and supplying a long-felt need'.[5]

For ETW, district nurses were a vital part of a public health system. He described them as 'the missing link' between the rich and the poor. 'There was no suspicion of pauperisation where [the district nurse] gave her help', he commented, 'and she could not be accused of patronage in any shape or form'.[6] The poor quickly welcomed the nurses into their homes in a way that simply was not possible with other roles or professions. Later, he summarised their unique contribution as follows:

> ... a district nurse must be much more than a nurse. It required something more than a kindly disposition for a trained nurse to go forth in all winds and weathers and in all circumstances amongst the lowest of the poor to do her nursing work. It was only because her heart was in her work that she did it, and this fact established a claim for the district nurse upon the respect and regard of the charitable. She had also to undertake great responsibilities. Unlike the hospital nurse, she had not a doctor always at her back. She had consequently to be self-reliant. She must know what to do - she must be a regular encyclopaedia of knowledge as to what was the proper treatment in sickness or in accident, and be prepared to act on any and every emergency. There was no limit to the possibilities of the usefulness of these nurses, and the good that they did could not be exaggerated.[7]

He also recognised that the district nurse could not act alone. 'There were three personages or classes of individuals concerned where district nursing was introduced', he observed, 'viz., the Committee, the doctor, and the nurse'.[8] Like a three-legged stool, if one component failed, the

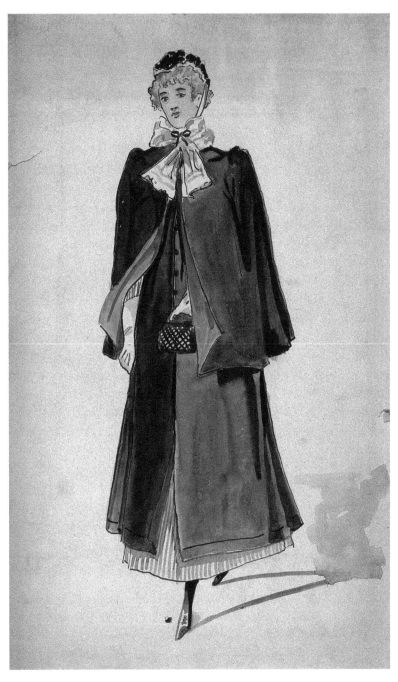

A district nurse with her outdoor uniform and bag.

whole system failed. To be successful, he stressed, each role should play its appropriate part.[9]

Despite its initial success, the Cheltenham Nursing Institution closed in October 1872 due to insufficient funding. Nevertheless, ETW returned to give his support in the 1880s to its successor, the District Nursing Association, which, he commented, became 'one of the most important and useful institutions in the town'.[10]

While ETW's thoughts were principally focused on supporting district nursing, in August 1868 he became embroiled in a troublesome case concerning the death of a flyman called Henry Dickenson. It was all part of being a medical practitioner where, at any time, one's professional judgement and reputation could be questioned under the glare of the public spotlight. The case had arisen after Dickenson was sent by his employer to the Lansdown cabstand and, later, died from what ETW believed to be an apoplectic fit. Mr Patterson, a Lansdown resident, discovered the unfortunate flyman when he drove back to his home, but was blocked by Dickenson's cab. After approaching the cab, Patterson found Dickenson 'apparently in a taste of stupor, whether from drunkenness or not'.[11] Then, taking the cab-horse by the rein to lead it out of the way, Dickenson fell forward on the footboard. Patterson immediately went to his assistance, and then his employer helped to take Dickenson home. It was here that he was attended by ETW. Sadly, he died the following day. The local press, keen to quash the 'absurd rumour' that Dickenson's death had resulted from a violent exchange with Patterson, had 'not the least shadow of a doubt' that there was anything untoward in this case. Consequently, it backed the holding of an inquest to corroborate ETW's assertion of the cause of death and avoid 'the committal of a gross and now inexcusable slander'.[12] The inquest was held on 2 August at the King William Inn,[13] where, given the considerable interest in the case, was packed to the rafters. There, ETW made the following statement:

> On Monday night shortly before 11 o'clock, I was called in to deceased at his home, 13, Victoria-place. I found him lying back in an armchair. I could not obtain any information what was the matter, except that be had been brought home in the state in which he then was - a state of insensibility. He appeared to be paralyzed. His mouth was open, his arms hanging down by his side, and his eyes closed. There was a pulse, neither particularly hard

nor slow. He was breathing quickly. My first impression was that the man had been drinking, but I could detect no indication of that. I opened the lids of his eyes, and placed a candle to them, and then saw that the pupils were set. My impression then was that he had had either a fit or a sunstroke. The extremities were warm. After being there about ten minutes, I gave instructions what to do, and left, intending to see him again next morning, but a person called before I had risen, and left word that the man had died in the night. In the course of the morning, I saw the body, I examined the head superficially, but noticed no bruises. I saw a few bruises on the shins, such that any man might have had - just a little discolouration. My impression before I came away - and it has been more confirmed since I have been in this room - was that the deceased was suffering from the effects of the sun, and that he died from the effects of exposure to the heat of it. Nothing I have heard is incompatible with that opinion. Sunstroke has the effect of causing the appearance of drunkenness.[14]

Further evidence was then given by the surgeon Dr Frederick Digby who, at the request of the deceased's friends, had examined the body. Digby claimed he found a mark on the throat, corresponding to the size of a thumb. He thought the mark may have been caused by a hand being placed on the throat, which might have led to apoplexy. Following this evidence, the coroner decided to adjourn the inquest so that another surgeon could undertake a post mortem examination. However, when they reconvened the jury heard that, because of the intense heat, the body had decomposed making it impossible to do a proper examination. Nevertheless, the independent surgeon commented that he did not consider that apoplexy had been caused by external pressure to the throat, and the jury came to the unanimous verdict that the flyman had died from natural causes.

While ETW found the case 'a rather annoying but at the same time amusing storm in a tea pot',[15] the controversy took a while to settle down. Around the same time, the Liberal-Conservative newspaper the *Cheltenham Times and Record* took a different view on the proceedings by claiming that the interest in the case had originally been excited through the following:

> ... a report – whether true or not we cannot say – which gained credence, that the medical man had taken the very unusual and questionable course

of writing to the Coroner direct, instead of first communicating with the police, to the effect that there was no necessity for holding an inquest, and the excitement became intensified by a very injudicious article which appeared in the *Examiner*, founded apparently by the evidence of one who had only seen the deceased for a few minutes on the night preceding his death.[16]

It now appeared that ETW was being put in the dock. Thankfully, as ETW later reflected it 'all ended in smoke' after 'a disreputable charge of manslaughter [had been] backed by a Dr Digby of evil reputation'.[17]

~~~

WHILE NOT DWELLING ON the flyman's case, ETW now became engrossed in quantifying the impact of the deficiency of water supply on the poorer districts of Cheltenham. Following drought conditions in August 1868 and a serious outbreak of typhoid, he made house visits to those parts of the town (Soho Place, Coach Road and Millbrook Street) situated on clay where he found that the poor were dependent on shallow wells and the water they could save from roofs. He reported:

> The state of the poor people was most deplorable. The shallow wells [are] dry, or yielding a most scanty supply, which had in most cases trickled from the dirty roof or from the still dirtier surface soil. Small pans of rain water were being hoarded with anxious care. Many had to go long distances for water to drink or make their tea. In more than one house no provision whatever was found for water; no well, no rain tub. What was required was begged where it could best be got, and the filthy waters of the Chelt were carried for miles and used almost universally at the lower part of the town for house purposes and washing.[18]

The picture he painted was of intolerable conditions in which pumps in porous soil were adjacent to 'middens and piggeries, with all their attendant filth'.[19] It was no wonder, he claimed, that 'the poor revolt from the nauseous draught, and beg the hill water day by day in the face of pains and penalties threatened by the Act of [the] local Water Company'.[20] He made a formal complaint to the Town Commissioners about the deplorable situation, and then engaged the public to review potential solutions to the problem through articulating the pros and cons of the five potential sources of water supply which Cheltenham had at its disposal. Firstly, he suggested, there were the hill springs: although they produced good quality water, nevertheless, it proved expensive to distribute, and so was unaffordable to the poor who would consider it a luxury. Then there were the springs in the town itself: although these could probably yield an inexhaustible supply, they had the disadvantage of being highly charged with minerals and so suited only for medicinal purposes. Water from the River Chelt was another possibility; but this was unsuitable because it was severely polluted. Alternative options included rainwater from catchment roof areas, but ETW considered this to be unpalatable in an urban area. He likened its colour to weak ink and its taste to that of soot; it was also a source that was both unreliable and difficult to store. The final potential solution came from the range of different wells which were supplied both by surface soakage and the River Chelt. However, these too were prone to contamination from sewer leakage and street washing.

Following ETW's complaint, the Town Commissioners responded by appointing a surveyor, who immediately corroborated ETW's claims, and then started negotiations with the Water Company and the owners of the properties to address how improvements could be made. Nevertheless, the negotiations failed, and a stalemate situation ensued. ETW concluded: 'The Occupiers cannot move. The Town Commissioners cannot move. The Water Company will not move. The owners will not move'.[21] ETW's frustration with Cheltenham's deficient water supply was to continue for years to come. For the time being, nothing could be done because the supply of hill water continued to rest in the hands of a trading company, whose interests differed from the Commissioners' and those who had the good of the town at heart.

~~~

DURING THIS PERIOD, THE Wilson family expanded further. On 15 October 1868, ETW was pleasantly surprised to hear that his first son Bernard was born with red hair. A second daughter, Helen, known as Nellie, followed just over a year later, this time appearing with brown hair. ETW also supported his brother Charly who had returned home in July

1865 after successfully completing the Ordnance Survey of Jerusalem, the city's first scientific mapping. The survey led to the creation of the Palestine Exploration Fund (PEF), and Charly was appointed its Chief Director for its proposed exploration of the rest of Palestine. To assist with fund-raising for the expedition, a meeting was held at the Assembly Rooms in Cheltenham on 16 November 1869, following which ETW was appointed as secretary to the Cheltenham PEF branch. It was an exciting project that would bring to life the secular aspects of the biblical narrative and ascertain the extent to which the scripture could be verified through archaeological evidence. 'We want to enable you', Charly said, 'to follow Christ in his travels through Palestine, David in his flight from Saul, and the Jewish armies in their movements over the country'.[22]

It was also a time when ETW advanced further in his profession. His election as a member of the widely-respected Metropolitan Association of Medical Officers of Health in 1867 was followed, less than two years later, by election onto the Gloucestershire branch's council of the British Medical Association (BMA), a position he was to hold for nearly forty years. Then, on 27 October 1870, he received the prestigious honour of becoming a Fellow of the Royal College of Physicians (FRCP) along with the distinguished London physician Charles Hilton Fagge (1838-83) and Henry Charlton Bastian (1837-1915), famous for his belief in archebiosis, the generation of living organisms from non-living matter. It was just reward for someone who had contributed recent papers on the subject of morphia injections, an advance he considered to be 'the greatest boon given to medicine since the discovery of chloroform',[23] as well as well-regarded research on sanitary issues.

7
The Fight against Infectious Diseases (1871-73)

Yellow fever plague in Buenos Aires – Plans for the Delancey Fever
Hospital – Use of disinfectants – Births of Pollie and Ted – Cheltenham
Sanitary Statistics second paper – Scarlet fever epidemic

*'During the autumn and winter Cheltenham was visited by a most malignant
epidemic of scarlet fever, very prevalent and very fatal from malignant sore
throat. I have never met with anything like it before or since'.*
~ ETW ~

A T THE BEGINNING OF 1871, the authorities in Buenos Aires, the
city of 'good air' - whose reputation as one of the healthiest places in
the world seemed unassailable - were becoming anxious. An outbreak of
yellow fever had occurred in one of the city's quarters. No precautionary
measures had been taken, and some doctors explicitly denied the facts to
avoid widespread panic. In February, the Carnival festivities only served
to accelerate the spread of the disease. By March, the monthly death toll
reached 11,000. A further 100,000 had fled from the city, while urgent
efforts were made to bury the dead amid reports that 'Men, supposed
dead, broke from their flimsy coffins on the way to the grave'.[1] One of
those caught up in the chaos was ETW's brother Harry. Following a severe
attack of scarlet fever in 1866, Harry had been advised to avoid English
winters and, in 1867, decided to travel to Argentina to become a farmer.[2]
Although he led a rough life close to the Indian frontier, he greatly enjoyed
the experience. It was noted:

[He was] fond of lassoing, and throwing the "bolas", and thought there
was nothing more exciting than having at the end of his lasso, buttoned on
to his saddle, a wild bull plunging about and bellowing, and often suddenly
charging him on his horse. It was in 1871, when lassoing some horses that
the lasso snapped, and recoiled with great force into his face, especially
damaging the right eye.[3]

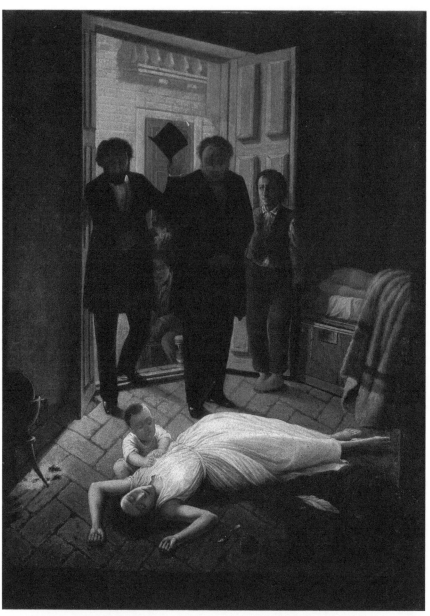

Yellow fever in Buenos Aires, 1871. Oil painting by Juan Manuel Blanes.

Afterwards, laid up in a Buenos Aires hospital with a seriously inflamed eye, he wrote to his brother as the epidemic raged all around. It was partly Harry's letters and partly two first-hand accounts (from a chaplain and a surgeon) which ETW used as source material for an article on the plague, later published in the *Food Journal*. His intent was to use the incident as a cautionary tale and share lessons learned about sanitary practice. 'Imagine a city', he implored, 'with narrow streets, crowded houses, and, in parts, a density of population almost beyond belief; where there is no provision for drainage beyond the cesspool or old well; [and] no water supply save that from the river - a river so poisoned by filth ...'.[4] Added to this, he remarked: 'Newly-made roads had been filled in with offal and refuse from the scavengers' carts before being macadamised, and these gave forth an almost intolerable stench after every shower of rain'.[5] It was only by accident or providence, ETW thought, that the city had avoided previous catastrophe. The causes of the epidemic were all too clear to him:

> ... decomposition of animal and vegetable matters of the vilest description, under an almost tropical sun, poisoned drinking supplies, densely crowded and filthy fever nests invited the outburst of epidemic disease, and fed it to the last; whilst an imperfect sanitary administration could but look on with dismay.[6]

Now, it was time for ETW to put into practice locally his specialist knowledge. On 12 April, after attending an important meeting at the General Hospital to take forward proposals to establish a fever hospital for the town, he was confirmed as one of the twelve trustees.[7] Provision for such a hospital was long overdue. Around twenty years earlier, soon after the General Hospital was opened, consideration had been made to adapt a small cottage in the grounds as a facility for isolating fever patients. However, the establishment of Cheltenham College in the immediate vicinity led the hospital authorities to abandon the idea out of politeness and consideration for such a prestigious institution. Then, in 1866, hopes of realising a fever hospital surfaced again when an eccentric local resident, Miss Susan Delancey, who lived in a suite of rooms at the Plough Hotel, told her doctor shortly prior to her death that she wished to bequeath £5,000 for this purpose. Nevertheless, given that her request was not written down, complications arose after her will was contested under the statute of mortmain. Despite this, three of the four legatees agreed to concur with Miss Delancey's wish on condition that the new hospital would bear her name. Other benefactors subsequently came forward, including the Revd J. H. Gabell, who contributed £1,000 to the purchase of a suitable 6-acre site at Pilley, in Leckhampton, for the hospital to be built.[8] Acting both as secretary to the trustees and as a member of the sub-committee charged with dealing with the building side of the project, ETW visited Bradford to inspect the newly-built fever hospital there and discuss the design proposals with the Bradford firm appointed for the Delancey project. Yet, implementation of the Bradford firm's design proved too costly. Therefore, it was later adapted by John Middleton, a local architect whom ETW knew from Friends in Council, in the hope that a more cost-effective option could be found.

In July, the scourge of disease hit close to home when Lily, Bernard and Nellie all contracted scarlet fever. Perhaps inspired by this event, ETW became determined to promote effective ways to curb the spread of infections. He spent several nights producing a small card on the use of

Disinfectants and How to Use Them.

By E. T. WILSON, B.M. Oxon., F.R.C.P. Lond., Physician to the Cheltenham General Hospital and Dispensary. In Packets of one doz., price 1s.

₊ The card will be found particularly suitable for heads of families, clergymen, and nurses; or for distribution among the artisans and tradesmen of our larger towns.

NOTICES OF THE PRESS.

" Mr. Wilson, who is a well-known medical officer, has placed upon a small card all the practical information necessary on the above subject. In addition, there are general directions when an outbreak of infectious disease occurs in a house. As these cards are obtainable for a shilling a dozen they should be widely circulated by philanthropic persons and sanitarians."— *The Metropolitan.*

"On the subject of disinfectants, the reader is referred to ' Disinfectants and How to use Them,' by Dr. Edward Wilson, of Cheltenham. The directions are printed upon cards, which are sold in packets of 12 for 1s , published by Mr. Lewis, 136, Gower Street. These cards should be in the possession of all medical practitioners, clergymen, and others, whose duty and desire it is to prevent, as much as possible, the spread of contagious diseases."—From Dr. Lionel Beale's Work on *Disease Germs,* 1872, p. 298.

" This little card is one of the most valuable aids in the diffusion of health knowledge that we remember to have seen. Clergymen, and all others interested in the welfare of the people, could not do a wiser thing than distribute them broadcast."—*Health.*

Advert for the card from a medical textbook, 1886

disinfectants which was later published by H.K. Lewis.[9] By 1903, 40,000 copies had been sold with many glowing reviews in the professional press attesting to its usefulness.[10] While ETW received no payment for it, he was simply gratified with the improved awareness it brought in the fight against infectious disease.

The following spring, as plans for the Delancey were potentially being blown off course, ETW's efforts became more focused on winning battles in the boardroom. In particular, he had many heated arguments with two of the trustees, whose ambition for delivering anything of lasting value seemed fairly modest. Fortunately, ETW could rely on support from William Henry Gwinnett (1809-91), a solicitor who acted as Treasurer to the Delancey Trust. 'If it had not been for the constant support of Mr Gwinnett', he commented, 'they might have had their way and the Hospital would have lost half its utility'.[11] Further delays ensued, following a rise in building costs, meaning that the final plans could only be agreed once guarantees were given that budgetary limits would not be exceeded. For this reason, an initial decision was made to build the smallpox block, with separate blocks for scarlet fever and diphtheria to follow later, once additional funds had been secured.

By the summer, ETW's attention became more directed to family life. Now sporting a moustache, 'by the advice if not the order'[12] of Mary, his off-spring increased to five following the birth of Edward Adrian on 23 July, and Mary Whishaw (known as Pollie), on 20 February, the previous year. ETW could never have predicted that the little red-haired boy he now welcomed into the world would later become 'our well loved 'Ted' of Antarctic fame'[13] who would become an explorer, natural historian, physician and artist.

On 6 August, ETW returned to the subject of Cheltenham's health when he presented his second paper on sanitary statistics, which he read before the BMA Meeting at Birmingham. His detailed analysis, which sought to determine the significant causes of death affecting the inhabitants of the different wards of the town, was well received. To support his findings, he drew a colour-coded map illustrating the complex interaction between those factors having greatest impact on the town's health. These included the different types of soil ('an important item, as controlling to a large extent the source of water-supply and sewage-soakage');[14] the position and extent of the main sewers (here, distinguishing between the old and modern ones); the nature of the water-supply, whether from the Water Company, the river, the wells, or rainwater; and the precise location of deaths, broken down by their cause, such as smallpox, diphtheria, scarlatina, or diarrhoea. Then, after adjusting the figures to take account of population and mortality statistics, he showed how the sewerage system and water-supply were the two most significant factors. While his analysis of the data revealed some important trends, it also raised unanswered questions. Why, for example, ETW wondered, did some children die from scarlatina in one street, whereas in neighbouring streets under similar conditions they made a full recovery? Why too did some children living in certain streets, invariably die before they were five? Further investigation was still needed. In the meantime, ETW concluded that Cheltenham's reputation as one of the healthiest places in the country would be best safeguarded through taking the following action: replacing its old sewers; providing wholesome water to the whole town, particularly the poorer quarters whose wells, owing to their location on sand-beds, were vulnerable to contamination; and isolating the first cases of any infectious disease. It was the last of these that was now urgently needed when, during the autumn and winter of 1872, Cheltenham was visited by a most malignant epidemic of scarlet fever, prompting the Town Commissioners to build a temporary fever hospital in the grounds of the Delancey. By the beginning of 1873, ETW was thankful that, after so many delays, building work for the proper hospital finally began. The day it could admit its first patient could not come soon enough.

8
Summary in St Petersburg (1873)

The Whishaw family – Hermitage – Vaccination – Hunting and fishing

'One day we went to the Foundling Hospital with its 800 babies under 6 weeks of age. They are drafted off to nurses in the country and we were told that only 20 per cent survive'.
~ ETW ~

MARY'S GRANDFATHER, WILLIAM WHISHAW (1746-1838), known to the family as 'Grandfather Speedwell' because of the colour of his eyes, was a merchant interested in shipping, who settled in St Petersburg *c*.1772 during Catherine the Great's reign. Mary herself had evidently impressed Tsar Nicholas II when she was introduced to him around the age of six.[1] Apart from being able to play the piano 'with Russian zest'[2] she also inherited her ability as an expert gardener through her grandfather's marriage to the Fock family.[3] Her father Bernhard Whishaw (1779-1868),[4] was an imposing figure, 6 feet tall with dark red hair, who became a senior partner in the trading firm Hills and Whishaw. He was full of integrity and showed great kindness, gentleness and generosity.[5] ETW knew the legendary stories about Bernhard's strength and endurance: how, during one tempestuous journey to Russia, his ship nearly sank, requiring him to hang onto the rigging for twenty-four hours; and another, where, at the age of seventy, he had walked 40 miles in the snow to complete a transaction in St Petersburg.[6] ETW must have thought that Mary had inherited some of her father's resilience, including when, around the age of nine, she had been taken on the perilous journey from St Petersburg to Cheltenham.

On 4 July, ETW and Mary sailed from Hull on the *SS Orlando*. The 260 feet-long 1500-ton iron screw steam ship completed the crossing to Gothenburg in around forty hours, the bright northern light allowing them to 'read the smallest print at midnight'.[7] Mary had last set foot in her birthplace St Petersburg twenty-three years earlier, but there was still a long way to go. Transferring by rail from Gothenburg to Stockholm, they boarded the *Aura* steamer which would accommodate them for the next four days through the Baltic as the ship weaved its way through the archipelago of low-lying islands, much inhabited with seals, to Abo (now Turku), Helsinki (then known as Helsingfors) and thence to Kronstadt, the port serving St Petersburg. Although the final leg of the journey, travelling north-west from St Petersburg, took them 12 miles along very bumpy roads, the final destination at Mourino, an estate belonging to Count Vorontsov-Dashkoff, proved idyllic. Here, the Whishaws and their English friends had settled comfortably in their luxurious wooden summer houses. It was in every sense 'a bit of England',[8] and 'a bright and comparatively care-free life [from where] visitors from the old country always carried away with them happy and perhaps somewhat envious recollections'.[9] ETW and Mary stayed with her brother Jim, once described as 'One of God Almighty's Noblemen'.[10] Jim was a keen bear-hunter; and it is possible that the *Boris the Bear-Hunter* (1895) adventure book, written by his nephew Fred Whishaw (1854-1934), who also settled in Cheltenham for a while, was inspired by Jim.[11] Universally known as 'charitable, generous, extremely simple-minded, haters of deceit or ostentation'[12] and blessed with a good sense of humour, the Whishaws made admirable hosts.

For ETW, one of the attractions of this holiday was the opportunity to visit the magnificent art collections at the Hermitage, probably founded in 1764 when Empress Catherine the Great acquired works from the Berlin merchant Johann Ernst Gotzkowsky. Nevertheless, after learning that the galleries were closed ETW's disappointment soon turned to relief upon discovering that 'a rouble note opens everything'[13] even though the intense heat in the city and the scorching pavements still made for uncomfortable sight-seeing.

ETW also used the visit to St Petersburg to develop his professional knowledge. Apart from visiting one of the city's hospitals,[14] whose separate entrances, he thought, were cleverly designed to enable three different types of infectious diseases to be isolated, he also visited the Foundling Hospital. Here, he was fascinated to learn about the successful practice of using calf-lymph for vaccinating against smallpox where, at times, as many as 200 vaccinations were being administered during a morning session.

Although compulsory vaccination had been introduced in the UK through the 1853 Vaccination Act, the current roll-out was not going smoothly. During the smallpox pandemic of 1870-75, for example, more than 13,000 deaths had occurred in 1871 in England and Wales alone.[15] In ETW's view, the current prevalence of smallpox was occurring through a combination of 'neglected and postponed vaccination' and 'the imperfect and insufficient manner in which vaccination [was] performed',[16] the latter, in particular, rekindling public apathy and widespread mistrust towards vaccination.

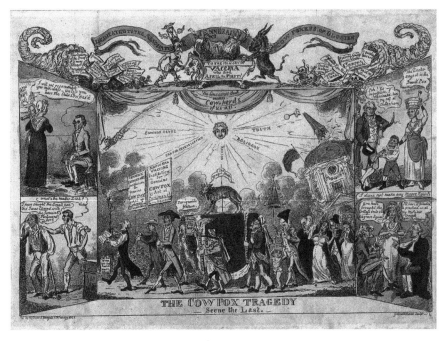

An attack on smallpox vaccination and on the Royal College of Physicians' advocacy of it. Coloured etching by G. Cruikshank, 1812.

Although calf lymph was used for a short time in the UK, during the 1840s, human lymph was the main source of the vaccine used from 1798 to 1881.[17] ETW noted that a Privy Council-commissioned report of 1869 previously rejected calf lymph on the grounds of some associated risks of failure and storage difficulties.[18] Yet, there were also significant problems in using human beings as vaccinifers, not least the risk of spreading infectious diseases such as syphilis. Now, at the Foundling Hospital, ETW arrived at a different conclusion. He heard from the doctor-in-charge Wilhelm Froebelius (1812-86) how vaccine from cows had been successfully used at the hospital since 1868, working side by side with lymph originally obtained from Edward Jenner.[19] To contribute to further medical discussion ETW recorded the process in detail:

> A heifer calf from two to four months old is taken every fourth day, the abdomen is cleanly shaved on a table specially adapted for the operation, and from 60 to 120 insertions are made in regular rows of from ten to fifteen pricks apiece. A light bandage is then applied, and the calf rejoins its companions in a clean and well-ventilated stable. On the fourth day the vesicles are ready; the lymph, however, is better on the fifth day, and none should be taken after the seventh. It is pressed from the vesicle by means of a small tenaculum; and I was assured that the effects were equally satisfactory whether the vaccination was performed in the summer or winter seasons.[20]

ETW was so impressed with the quality of the vaccine that he brought some of the lymph back to Cheltenham, transporting it in capillary tubes, where it was used to great success at the public vaccine station, producing well-developed vesicles.[21] Later, he urged the Government to reconsider using animal vaccine lymph whose supply, he stressed, 'should be practically inexhaustible, and at the same time above suspicion'.[22] In 1879 the Government decided to set up an Animal Vaccine Station and, two years later, started to produce calf lymph on a large scale. Under the Vaccination Act of 1898 calf lymph (in glycerinated form for preservation) became the standard vaccine in England.[23] While the change in policy was not all down to ETW's efforts, nevertheless it shows the sound medical judgement that he exercised.

For the rest of their stay, ETW and Mary were able to relax and enjoy rural life in Russia. For ETW, there was time for fishing for trout on the mosquito-infested River Zaritch and for hunting, begun at 4 a.m. to avoid the suffocating heat. While they failed to catch sight of bear, elk, lynx or wolves, they often spotted the tracks of bear on the search for ants' nests as the party swept through the vast forests, precariously perched on a tarantass (a springless four-wheeled horse-drawn carriage used in Russia). Another day's shooting was spent at Ostromancha,[24] about 20 miles from Mourino, near Lake Lagoda.

During the long journey home, they stopped in Stockholm which they considered 'a fairy city' populated by people incorporating 'a delightful mixture of English stolidity with French politeness'.[25] After visiting the city museum's displays of flints, bronze and evidence of Neolithic Man in Scandinavia, they crossed Sweden via the inland lakes and the Trolhättan Canal, taking in views of the famous Trolhättan falls. After a rough crossing in heavy seas along Dogger Bank, they eventually arrived back in Cheltenham on 11 August. While there was much of enduring interest for ETW from this trip, on this occasion it was Mary who read a paper about her Russian experiences for the Ladies' Friends in Council which she had helped to establish in 1872.

9

'My greatest work' (1874-81)

Delancey Board of Trustees – Smallpox Block – Expansion of family
– Move to *Westal* – Museum work – Eccentric and famous patients –
Scarlet Fever Block

*'No one will ever know the difficulties which attended the early meetings of
the Delancey Trustees. Little was known of sanitary matters, still less of fever
hospitals. There were very few in the country and most of these only fit for
cattle – utterly unsuited to human beings'.*
~ ETW ~

ON 18 APRIL 1874, as part of the celebrations for their wedding
anniversary, ETW and Mary travelled to Gloucester. They went to
witness the drama of the Severn Bore pushing back against the river's
flow. 'The river, which was flowing gently towards the sea', the *Globe*
commented, 'was in a moment reversed in its course, and rushed up
a mass of waters, some feet in height, throwing mud and water high
in the air'.[1] ETW knew all about pushing against the flow. For almost
the last three years he had been at loggerheads with certain factions
on the Delancey Board of Trustees. There were several elderly men,
who brought narrow-minded and antiquated views to the table. In one
case, it led to a permanent estrangement with a fellow physician.[2] The
situation was made worse by the lack of support from Clement Hawkins,
the senior surgeon at the General Hospital. While Hawkins refused to
join the trustees, ETW noted that he 'used all his influence to cut down
the plans for the buildings'.[3] ETW felt it was only through support from
other trustees, such as W.H. Gwinnett, the Revd J.H.L. Gabell,[4] J. T. Agg-
Gardner, and Dr J. Abercrombie, that he succeeded in providing 'anything
more than wooden sheds, or very inferior and scanty brick buildings for
the town'.[5]

As ETW watched the bore's energy dissipate and the river's water
return to a gentle-flowing harmonised state, he could perhaps reflect that
his own energies were now being channelled towards positive outcomes as

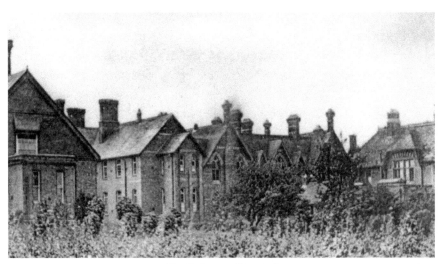

The Delancey Hospital

the finishing touches were being made to the first phase of the Delancey Hospital. Two months later, on 15 June, the formal opening ceremony for the Smallpox Block took place. The one-storey-high building, built of red coral bricks, with black bands, and a dark-brown tile roof, contained fourteen beds, a nurse's room, a small surgery, and a kitchen. Inside, the spacious rooms were well-ventilated, using rods and cranks to open the windows inwards, and were decorated with white-glazed bricks, used to promote cleanliness. A disinfecting room was located in the basement, and there was provision for a drying shed and a small mortuary. After the Revd Canon Bell, standing in for the Lord Bishop of the diocese, completed the opening ceremony, it was ETW's contribution that was singled out for the highest praise. The Conservative Party politician Sir Alexander Ramsay, 3rd Baronet (1813-75), described ETW's efforts simply as a labour of love. Likewise, ETW considered the Delancey Hospital to be his 'greatest work in Cheltenham'.[6] He commented:

> ... altho financially its erection has been due to Miss Delancey, Mr Gabell, Mr Charles Wilson [no relation to ETW] and many others, the plan was essentially my own worked out with great care and after obtaining all the help I could find from Hospitals already built - and applying it to the special needs of Cheltenham and its neighbourhood.[7]

ETW appreciated that the need for fever hospitals might, one day, come to an end in the light of new antitoxin discoveries and the delivery of preventative services but, for now, was confident that their use would be fully justified. As the year drew to a close, he proudly penned the hospital's first annual report. Since opening on 15 July, eight cases of smallpox had been treated. On each occasion, the interventions had stopped potential epidemics, leading the trustees 'to claim that "the Delancey Hospital has, so far, fully carried out the anticipations of its promoters, and has earned the generous support of the inhabitants of Cheltenham and its neighbourhood"'.[8] In the longer term, the trustees' planning assumptions for the smallpox block also proved to be correct. While they were initially criticised for making provision for only ten beds, considered by many to be 'absurdly small for the purpose intended',[9] their strategy was shown to be effective, even when faced with a serious epidemic that had broken out in Gloucester and threatened to spill over to Cheltenham. The risks were managed partly through building an annexe to the smallpox block to cope with any peak demand, and partly through enlisting local support from medics and the wider community to ensure that the very first cases were

immediately treated as soon as they appeared. By adopting this approach, ETW considered Cheltenham to be 'the safest town in England'[10] when it came to smallpox treatment. The figures during his management of the hospital bear out how effective the treatment was (see Appendix 3).

No sooner was the first phase completed than ETW started to plan for the construction of the second phase, the Scarlet Fever, or Scarlatina Block. 'What has been done for smallpox is undoubtedly possible, though far more complex, in the case of scarlatina', he wrote in a letter to the *Cheltenham Examiner*.[11] As current treatment then relied on the use of small

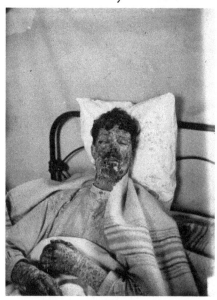

Gloucester smallpox epidemic, 1896, Edwin Davis, a smallpox patient.
Photograph by H.C.F., 1896.

sanatoria, ETW recognised that these could become breeding grounds for
the infection itself, given that patients were not isolated there. Promoting
the need for the local community to unite in combatting this threat and
erect a building for scarlatina patients, he commented:

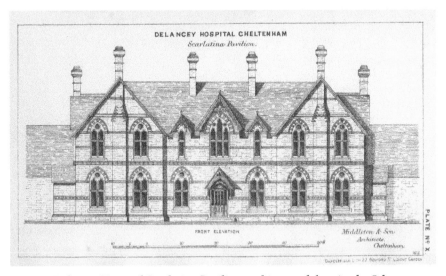

*Delancey Hospital Scarlatina Pavilion, architectural drawing by John
Middleton.*

The advantages of such a building can scarcely be over-rated. The rooms,
specially adapted for the treatment of the sick, would themselves promote
recovery, while the facilities afforded for effectual isolation of the patient
and the thorough disinfection of all that belongs to him, would encourage
a hope that epidemics might be cut short at their onset. The experiment
has never been fairly tried with scarlatina; let Cheltenham lead the way.[12]

~~~

DURING THIS PERIOD THE Wilson family was still growing, both
in number and eminence, with ETW's mounting reputation as a
physician. Both led to the requirement for a larger house. In September
1874, just after their fourth daughter Jessie (Jessica Frances) was born,
they moved around the corner to *Westal* on Montpellier Parade. *Westal*
(its site now covered by the Eagle Tower car park) was a large, detached

'Regency' house, with a private carriage sweep, large gardens and stabling, greenhouses and ferneries, marble fire places, four reception rooms, ten bedrooms, a nursery and servants' quarters. The requirements of the household meant that five servants were employed in the house alone - not untypical of the period. Tragically, Jessie's life was short-lived. Less than five months after celebrating the arrival of a fifth daughter, Ida Elinor, on 20 September 1875, the family mourned Jessie's loss when she died of tubercular disease of the brain.

~~~

D URING THE EARLY PART of 1875, ETW provided some assistance to Cheltenham College Museum. Established in 1870, the museum had become an important attraction for the town after being opened to the public on 31 January 1871. Until a proper public museum building could be established, it acted as a substitute repository for local artefacts. Here, he helped Charles Pierson[13] to arrange some Neolithic human skulls

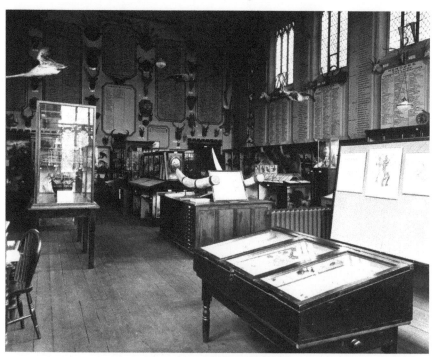

Cheltenham College Museum.

discovered during the 1863-5 excavations of Belas Knap Long Barrow, near Winchcombe. Throughout his life ETW championed the use of museums, and always took care to ensure that any artefacts of national importance he acquired were donated to the most appropriate institution. Later on, for example, he received a preserved specimen of a fowl's ovaries containing an egg *in situ*. Its interest stemmed from the fact that it had been prepared and mounted by Dr Edward Jenner (1749-1823). The specimen was originally given to the physician John Baron (1786–1851), who lived in Cheltenham during his retirement and wrote a biography of Jenner. It was subsequently passed to Dr Baron's sister and then to Dr John Abercrombie, before being given to ETW.[14] He then arranged for it to donated to the Hunterian Museum at the Royal College of Surgeons.

~~~

LATER, ON 12 JULY, ETW noted 'a queer experience' when Colonel Robert Knox Trotter (1807-76) died in a house, a nursing home at that time, opposite *Westal*. Trotter was a close associate of France's last monarch, Napoleon III (1808-73), also known as Louis-Napoleon. After the emperor was imprisoned at the fortress of Ham, following a failed *coup d'état* at Boulogne in 1840, it is thought that Trotter assisted his escape on 25 May 1846. A humorous cartoon recorded the event. It shows Napoleon disguised as a workman wearing wooden clogs and a smock, accompanied by his doctor, Dr Henri Conneau (1803-77), and a man in military uniform, nonchalantly walking past the guard. When Napoleon died in 1873 it was Dr Conneau who embalmed his body. According to ETW, Colonel Trotter had also requested that his body be embalmed. ETW commented:

> As Dr. Conneau had done [the embalming of the emperor] and was a friend of the family he was invited to do the same in this instance – and I thus had the pleasure of seeing something of the man who had so bravely aided his master to escape from the fortress of Ham.[15]

The Trotter incident was one of several that ETW recalled involving various eccentric or famous patients during his long career in a town much favoured as a retirement resort by former colonial members and military officers. One of his most eccentric was George Perton (c.1801-81),[16] a

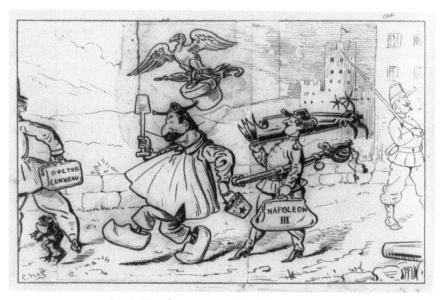

Louis-Napoleon escaping from Ham in 1846.

Birmingham businessman who came to retire in Cheltenham, living at Prestbury Mansion. A member of the Birmingham Stock Exchange, Perton had accrued vast wealth through manufacturing jewellery, paper, pens and iron. ETW recalled having consultations in Perton's brass-mounted chariot, during which he produced voluminous notes on all his symptoms over the preceding weeks. When ETW wrote him a prescription Perton invariably commented, 'Now remember no water, we can get it cheaper in Prestbury'.[17] It seems likely that they would also have discussed their love of art, Perton having collected some old master paintings, including works by Palamedes, Bruegel, and Canaletto. At the time of his death, Perton's estate was worth nearly £300,000, £400 of which was bequeathed to ETW. The following year, ETW noted another unusual experience with one of his patients, Maria Middleton, the wife of the architect John Middleton (1820-85). He wrote:

> In the early days of the Telephone a wire was laid from the pulpit in Christchurch to Mrs Middleton's bedroom where we often had the pleasure of criticising the sermon as the preacher proceeded.[18]

Another of ETW's noteworthy patients was Prince Alemayehu Tewodros (1861-79), the son of the Ethiopian emperor Tewodros II. The child prince, whose ancestry could be traced back to King Solomon and the Queen of Sheba, became orphaned in April 1868; his father, unwilling to accept defeat during the British conquest of Magdala in the Abyssinian campaign, committed suicide, and his mother died from an illness. Having been captured in the aftermath of the battle, Alemayehu was made a ward of Queen Victoria, and, in 1870, sent to Cheltenham and, later, to Rugby to receive a public-school education. When he died from pleurisy in 1879 at the age of nineteen, ETW commented: 'He was a nice lad and joined in all the games of an English playground with zest and success'.[19] In contrast, Queen Victoria made the following comment in her journal:

> It is too sad! All alone, in a strange country, without a single person or relative, belonging to him .... His, was no happy life, full of difficulties of every kind, and he was so sensitive, thinking people stared at him on account of his colour, that I fear he would never have been happy.[20]

~~~

IN OCTOBER 1876, ETW was saddened by the death of Dr Henry Rumsey (1809-76), one of the great experts of his day on public health and one of ETW's closest friends in Cheltenham.[21] ETW commented, 'He had done an immense amount of Sanitary work without fee or reward save empty honour of which there was plenty'.[22] Two years earlier, following Rumsey's ill health, ETW had arranged a testimonial for him compiled by Rumsey's friends. ETW added:

> His rare talents and special ability in sanitary matters were appreciated by the few but were scarcely known or recognised in his own locality – nor were the utilities by the Government as they certainly ought to have been.[23]

~~~

AS THE SCARLET FEVER Block, also known as the Gabell Block (after the benefactor the Revd Gabell), was nearing completion, ETW focused his attention on completing the furnishing requirements in time for open days, held from the end of March 1877, prior to its formal opening. The two-storey building, constructed in a similar style to the Smallpox Block, comprised seven private wards on the ground floor and two on the upper. Each initially accommodated three beds, but could cope with an expansion to eight. It also included a large convalescents' room. Further expansion was possible through the addition of wings at either end. The *Cheltenham Examiner* reporter described it as 'a marvel of hospital construction', commenting:

> ... throughout the building no precaution against the spread of infection seems to have been neglected, no appliance for the provision of that great desideratum, pure air, to have been overlooked, and nothing which could minister to the comfort or pleasure of the patients, to have escaped attention.[24]

Whilst smallpox could be eradicated almost entirely, largely helped through people's fear of the disease and wish to isolate themselves from it immediately, scarlet fever proved more problematic because of its potential to be spread through the most unlikely of channels. Drawing on his own experience, ETW commented:

> ... our water and our milk may be boiled, but who shall guarantee that scarlet fever scales are not sent to us in our newspapers, that fever-stricken children have not been sitting on the clothes sent in by our tailor; or that the tradesman who serves us has not a moment before been at the bedside of an infected child.[25]

Moreover, the disease was not always taken seriously because of the widespread use of the term 'scarlatina' to refer to mild cases of the disease. ETW recognised that those cases were, in fact, as infectious as more pronounced cases. Later, to support this view, he showed that only thirty cases, or 1.5 per cent, had proved fatal out of the total of 1,804 cases that had been treated between 1877, when the scarlet fever block was first used, and 1898, even though many of these had been some of the worst cases he had ever seen. Additional figures bear out the effective treatment provided by the hospital (see Appendix 3). Another advantage of providing separate accommodation for the treatment of scarlet fever arose from the tendency of convalescing patients' skin to peel. ETW stressed:

[This] was the most infectious part and most infectious time, and if it were allowed to go through its course in a private house, this infectious material, which had a vitality [one] could hardly credit, would become hidden in all the crooks and crannies, ready to issue forth and attack all who came within its reach.[26]

Therefore, he advised patients to be sent to the Delancey where the interior design of the building, with its rounded angles and corners and use of disinfectants, helped to eradicate any places where infection might lurk. While ETW recognised that there were no social boundaries in terms of who could become infected by the disease, he attributed the significant immunity of Cheltenham's upper classes from scarlet fever entirely to the hospital's 'prompt isolation...of cases which arose from time to time in the lower parts of the town'.[27]

While the town now appeared to be relatively safe from the scourge of smallpox and scarlet fever, further effort was needed if the trustees' vision was to be realised to also cater for diphtheria patients. However, more time was needed before ETW could put this final piece of the jigsaw in place.

10
A Sense of Déjà Vu (1878-84)

'The battle of the waters' – District nursing and the Charity
Organisation Society – *Sunnymede* – Protest against Anti-Vaccination –
Galton prize

'... *if we do not do something both to use and spread the knowledge we possess,
I fear our consciences will not acquit us of all blame*'.
~ ETW ~

A T THE START OF 1878, ETW was becoming increasingly frustrated
with the inaction of the authorities to stem the spread of disease
through an inadequate water supply. Fifteen months earlier, he had given
a talk entitled 'Practical hints on health' to the Young Men's Christian
Association (YMCA), in which he spoke about Cheltenham's vulnerability
to water pollution. As the town was located on porous soil, water became
trapped after seeping down to a layer of impervious clay. Because of this,
he cautioned, well-water, filled with soakings from streets, gutters, drains
and sewers, was never safe to drink unless it was boiled. Comparing the
town's annual mortality rate of 20 per 1,000 with sixty-four other districts
in England, where the equivalent average ranged between 15 and 17, he
concluded that there were at least 200 preventable deaths in Cheltenham
every year. He questioned:

> Are we not in some measure answerable to them? – for these 200 lives
> sacrificed year by year, victims to neglect of nature's laws - if we do not do
> something both to use and spread the knowledge we possess, I fear our
> consciences will not acquit us of all blame.[1]

A clean water supply was of such critical importance, he felt, that it
should be debated as one of the key issues in local elections. Bad water, he
recognised, also led to problems of drunkenness and alcoholism as men
were often driven to pubs to drink something more palatable. In March
1878, he was able to raise his concerns in the Houses of Parliament. The

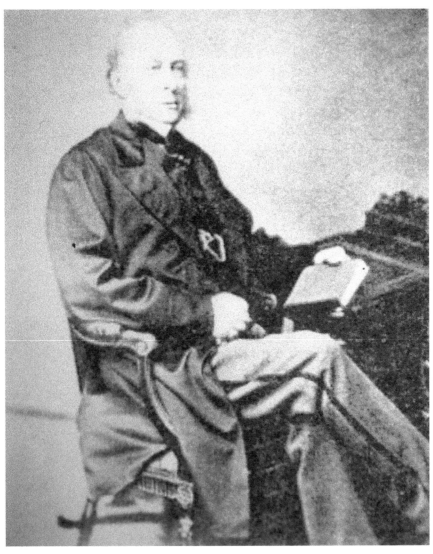

Dr Thomas Wright, Cheltenham's first Medical Officer of Health

question of whether the River Severn could be used as a suitable supply of drinking water for Cheltenham, potentially providing the town with a practically limitless supply, was once again discussed. In a remarkably similar re-run of their first appearance as expert witnesses in front of the House of Commons committee, ETW and Dr Thomas Wright, this time acting in the capacity of Cheltenham's Medical Officer of Health, opposed the Cheltenham Water Company's Bill on behalf of the Town

Commissioners. Once again, they used photographic evidence to demonstrate the existence of fungus caused by sewage contamination in the tanks of Severn water at Worcester.

In April, the full saga of the controversy was cleverly captured in 'The battle of the waters - a legend', an amusing parody of Henry Wadsworth Longfellow's 'The Song of Hiawatha' (1855). Published anonymously in the *Cheltenham Examiner*, the verse was supposedly penned by ETW's friend James Winterbotham.[2] It told the story of an innocent and harmless Indian, TSHELT-NUM-WARTA KUMPNEE, who was robbed by a dishonest, greedy giant called KAW-PAW-AYSHEN. Of particular relevance to the evidence that ETW gave to the House of Commons committee was the debate about whether the River Severn comprised wholesome water or was polluted with sewage:

Then they lifted up their voices,
KAW-PAW-AYSHN did and KUMPNEE
Very loudly cried and clamoured
Loudly KAW-PAW called for water
Loudly KUMPNEE praised the Sewage
Both proclaimed the wrongs and dangers
Told in their own way the stories
(Very different were their stories)
Called for aid to the KUMITY
Made them weary with their stories
Day by day with ceaseless calling
Called their men of facts and figures
Called their men of fears and fancies
Brought them from the banks of rivers
From the ancient seats of learning
Brought them from the crowded City
From the sleepy streets of small towns
Brought Geologists and Doctors
Aldermen and Mayors and Barons
Chemists Architects and Bargees
Lock-men, Schoolmasters and Bankers
Old J.P.'s and youthful C.E.'s,
LL. D.'s and F.R.S.'s,

Men who never tasted water
Men who nothing else had tasted
Men of Germs and Men of No-germs
Men of Theory, Men of Practice
Men who liked the Sewage-water
Men who didn't seem to do so
(Very different were their stories)
But the simple truths of KUMPNEE
Of the witnesses of KUMPNEE
Fell unheeded upon KAW-PAW
Prejudiced and headstrong KAW-PAW,
Not the least convinced would he be
Even when the wondrous witness
HAWK-HIS-LIE the wondrous witness
(Kindly wishing to convince him
Not to mention the KUM-ITY)
Unto many a simple question
Spoke in answer twenty minutes
Telling all the wondrous story
Of the sweetness of the River,
How if you put in a dead cat
Nasty-smelling, dead a fortnight,
Bloated, swollen, quite revolting,
If you put it in the River
(Hundreds frequently were found there)
Ere two miles it would have travelled
(Half an hour 'twould take to do it)
Lo! You found it sweet and wholesome
You might stir it in your liquor
Find it not the least unpleasant
No! he pledged his word upon it
'Twould be fragrant as a nosegay
(Every day's experience showed it).
Just the same it was with Sewage.
Let a town of fifty thousand
Pour their Sewage in the River
Let it flow the magic two miles

Lo! 'Twas harmless, pure and pleasant
Not a trace of filth was left there
'Twas the best of drinking water
"Yes, I pledge my word upon it
Nothing nasty can be left there
It is all burnt up and done for,
Just as if't had never been there –
It is oxidized, your Lordship,
Oxidized the Chemists call it".[3]

In giving his evidence, ETW opposed the case by 'HAWK-HIS-LIE the wondrous witness'. Thomas Hawksley (1807-93) was the leading hydraulic engineer of the nineteenth century who personally supervised around 150 water-supply projects, including the Severn scheme. ETW told the Committee that the Severn was unfit as a source of supply for drinking water if something better could be obtained; this was because of its inherent impurity and its use for transporting goods. Not only did it receive sewage from a large population but also, he thought, its sewage would not be oxidised as Hawksley had suggested. ETW made his views clear:

> In case of an epidemic upon the stream, he [ETW] should not like to trust a run of twenty miles as destroying the danger of infection. Even if there was anything in [Hawksley's] theory, and an epidemic raged in Worcester, a passing barge might drop the source of the infection at the very mouth of the intake. Analysis would not show if water was medically affected.[4]

ETW also told the Committee about his pioneering research on sanitary statistics, which showed the relation of disease to water supply and linked high rates of mortality to inadequate water supply in the poorer parts of the town. Quoting specific cases, he provided evidence that he had arrested diarrhoea by merely changing the water supply of the patient, while in the case of the inhabitants of Millbrook Street, who were without water, he found typhoid in nine out of thirteen houses.

After several days of the hearing, the Company's Bill was defeated; nevertheless, a rival Bill, put forward by the Town Commissioners, successfully led to the acquisition of the Company's works. While this avoided the immediate risk of pollution from the Severn, significantly, it also made provision for supplementing the supply of spring water by mixing it with river water should this be required in future. The fact that Tewkesbury's inhabitants were now drinking water from the River Severn with seemingly few ill-effects started to polarise medical and scientific opinion on the matter.

While ETW could be forgiven for feeling a sense of *déjà vu* regarding his quest for clean drinking water, the same was also true for the provision of district nursing in Cheltenham. In 1864, it had been his suggestion that led to the creation of the Cheltenham Nursing Institution, which provided a system of district nursing for the sick poor. Fifteen years later, on 18 June 1879, his interest in establishing a Charity Organization Society (COS) for the town also stemmed from his desire to provide district nursing. The *Cheltenham Examiner* reported:

> Dr. Wilson ... spoke of the desirability of the society to be formed becoming not only the centre for private benevolence, but also connected with all the charitable institutions of the town, so that no one person might be receiving aid from many of those institutions at the same time, as had not been infrequent hitherto. He thought also it would be a great boon to the town if a system of trained nurses to attend the poor could be established, after the example set at Liverpool.[5]

Of all the institutions with which he was connected throughout his career, it was the District Nursing Association that he considered gave him 'most satisfaction and pleasure'.[6] From ETW's perspective, the benefits that nursing could bring were considerable. Apart from being able to meet the poor's needs with much greater certainty he also recognised the following:

> The trained nurse will bring valuable and skilled aid in carrying out the directions of the medical attendant, in promoting a better hygiene and general cleanliness, in assisting and superintending simple cooking for the sick, in giving warning of impending danger, and, when necessary, urging isolation or removal, in cases of infectious disease, to the Delancey Hospital ....[7]

ETW highlighted further benefits. For the clergy and benevolent people in general, the nurses could draw 'their attention to the actual wants of poor people, without the risk of deception and fraud'.[8] For medical professionals, the nurses would perform minor operations and lend patients any necessary equipment. For the public, they would provide early warning to counter the spread of infectious diseases. For public bodies and Medical Officers of Health, the network of trained nurses would highlight and fix defects in the system. By the end of 1880, ETW was pleased to report that the association already employed a lady superintendent and 'two thoroughly-trained and efficient nurses who had already made themselves most acceptable in many houses for the poor'.[9] Despite this success, additional funding was needed to sustain and expand the services; this was a challenge that ETW now sought to address.

~~~

D URING THIS PERIOD, FURTHER additions were made to the family. Elsie Violet was born on 3 June 1878, later suffering from mental health problems, and then, on 29 January 1881, James Vernon. Known as 'Father Jim', he became a priest in the Catholic Crusade, which combined high Anglo-Catholicism and Marxist-Socialist politics. ETW described him as 'a rare good fellow'.[10] From 1878, ETW started the annual tradition at home of playing Father Christmas, usually appearing after being called away on 'an urgent medical emergency'. It added fun to what was always a particularly important family occasion for the Wilsons. In January 1881, however, ETW noted that a real emergency occurred when Cheltenham experienced one of the most severe snowstorms in recent years. He commented:

> ... [the snow] drifted to a level with the College railings along by the Northwick Gallery. Ladies slept at the Hospital after the ball being unable to get any further and I had to wade through snow up to my middle in finding my way to Westholme where Mrs Middleton was lying ill.[11]

It was also a time when the family got into country habits. From September 1879, Mary rented a little farm, *Sunnymede*,[12] (no longer extant, site originally located near Wards Road, Up Hatherley) on the outskirts of Cheltenham. Here she bred poultry and practised 'scientific farming', whilst the children kept farmyard pets. She was the first to import and breed Plymouth Rocks from America and became the author of the *ABC of Poultry* (1880), which was considered a definitive work for many years. Much of the farm produce was consumed in the household or sold in the local area, although it was never very profitable. The farm produced over forty varieties of apples and pears, amongst other crops, which were often shown in local agricultural shows. It was not all plain sailing; on 7 July 1884 ETW noted that Mary lost forty-six prize chickens from a coop. A policeman was called but it was soon found to be the work of a fox. Mostly, however, the farm and its produce were a source of great pleasure and pride.

On the medical professional front, it also proved to be a fulfilling time. At meetings of the National Association for the Promotion of Social Science (NAPSS) ETW read papers on the subjects of 'Fever Hospitals' and, in October 1878, 'Isolation as a means of arresting Epidemic Disease'. At this last meeting, held in Cheltenham, he made a strong case for further investment into isolation hospitals and provided practical pointers to resolving many of the complex issues associated with them. He also called for a Government Board of Health inquiry into isolation hospitals to improve central coordination and establish basic facts about their provision. In the absence of such data, he resorted to presenting the results of his own state-of-the-art survey based on information he collected from 128 UK hospitals.[13] For ETW, isolation hospitals' services were as essential as those provided by the police and fire brigade: while the latter suppressed riots and flames, the hospitals extinguished disease before it got out of control. Inspired by a picture of Captain Shaw, famous for introducing modern methods into the Metropolitan Fire Brigade, being surrounded by wires connecting him to all parts of the city, ETW imagined:

... officers presiding over the health of that great city, sitting with ambulances and staff in attendance for the first telegraphic intimation of a case of typhus or small-pox, ready to convey it at once to a place of safety and to stamp out all traces of the disease.[14]

During the Cheltenham meeting ETW entertained the epidemi-ologist William Farr (1807-83), regarded as one of the founders of medical statistics. The following month, not long after moving his practice from a room in The Priory to a more central location, at 13 Cambray,[15] he was elected as President of the Gloucestershire Branch of the BMA. One of the immediate priorities in this new role was to promote vaccination. In Cheltenham, Baron de Ferrieres, the local Liberal Party candidate for the 1880 General Election, stirred up a local debate on this through promising, if elected, to repeal the Compulsory Clauses of the Vaccination Act.[16] A month later, he went further, amending his stance towards a total repeal of the Act.[17] ETW heartily encouraged the medical profession to protest against the Anti-vaccinationists. Nevertheless, it proved a difficult argument to win. The case against vaccination was promoted strongly by the physician Sir Isaac Pennington (1745-1817), who promulgated the following story about Dr Edward Jenner, the discoverer of vaccination for smallpox, when Jenner resided in Cheltenham:

> ... he [Pennington] publicly stated that although Dr. Jenner recommended the practice to others, yet he was personally distrustful of it, and had abandoned it in his own family.[18]

Despite this being refuted by a pro-vaccinator, who published a letter[19] from Jenner confirming the inaccuracy of Pennington's statement, ETW and many of his medical colleagues were disappointed when the Baron was successfully elected as the town's M.P. Nevertheless, their fears were soon allayed when the new Liberal Government omitted to introduce their controversial Bill.

A little over a year later, on 16 June 1881, ETW had a more enjoyable task when he helped to steward one of the most prestigious events that had been held at the Assembly Rooms for many years. The occasion was the Midland Union of Natural History Societies' 'Conversazione';[20] this provided a fascinating range of displays, including specimens of archaeology, botany, conchology, entomology, geology, geometry, microscopy, ornithology, physics, and physiology. While ETW showed some examples of his photomicrography, practical demonstrations were also being given of recent inventions such as microphones, spectroscopes, and telephones. Further intellectual stimulation followed in July when he met Charles-Édouard Brown-Séquard (1817-94), the Mauritian physiologist and neurologist who gave his name[21] to paralysis caused by

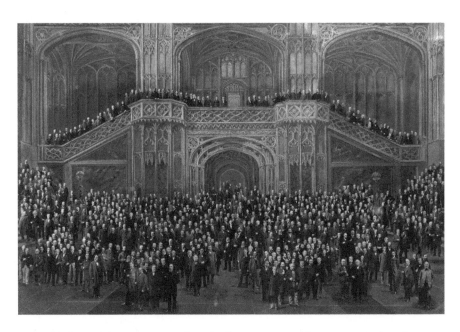

*Members of the International Medical Congress, London, 1881, Herbert Rose
Barraud, and detail (below) showing ETW (with arm crossed).*

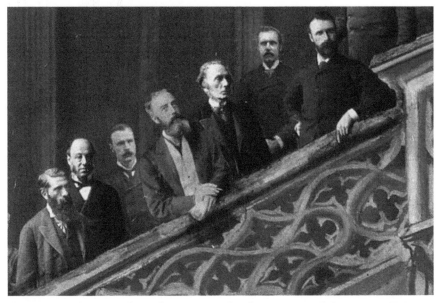

damage to the spinal cord. Then, at the beginning of August, ETW was
thrilled to attend the Seventh International Medical Congress, held at St

James's Hall, London, where he heard the opening address of Sir James Paget (1814-99) as President and saw the Prince of Wales, the future King Edward VII. More than 3,000 delegates attended the event, 684 of which, including ETW, were captured in an extraordinary composite group photograph.

~~~

I N FEBRUARY 1883, ETW's brother Charly left Egypt, where he had been serving on a special mission under the British consul-general to counter the Egyptian nationalist uprising led by Arabi Pasha (1839-1911). His intention was to resume his duties as Director of the Ordnance Survey in Ireland on 1 April. ETW fondly recalled visiting him during a family holiday in Ireland in 1877, shortly after Charly started his new position. They had met in his office in Phoenix Park, Dublin, and then toured through the scenic Wicklow countryside and along the River Dargle. Since then, Charly had been created K.C.M.G. in 1881 for services in Asia Minor and Eastern Rumelia, had been promoted to brevet colonel on 19 April 1883 and, two months later, made an Honorary D.C.L. of Oxford. ETW was under no illusion that his brother would not remain desk-bound for long.

In the early part of 1884, ETW compiled data on the relevant pedigrees of the Wilson and Whishaw families; this formed part of a study on genetic inheritance conducted by the eminent Victorian polymath Francis Galton (1822-1911), who coined the phrase 'nature versus nurture'.[22] It was a subject that fascinated ETW throughout his life.[23] In June, Galton awarded ETW a prize of £7 for one of the best submissions received. In the study, among the bodily strength features that ETW had recorded for Charly were 'great powers of endurance' and 'energy great in certain directions', while his character and temperament were summarised as 'Passionate but well under control – nervous but with great determination – retiring'.[24] Little did ETW know that his brother's personal qualities were soon to be tested to the limit.

11
'Too late – too late!' (1885)

Death of General Gordon – Seeking a scapegoat – Defending Charly's
reputation

*'... the telegrams at the club were closely and eagerly scanned during the
stirring times of the battles in the desert and the fight for the Nile – Alas that
was all in vain – Too late – too late!'*[1]
~ ETW ~

IN THE EARLY HOURS of 26 January 1885, the rebellious forces under
the leadership of the Mahdi broke into the fortified city of Khartoum,
which had laid under siege for nearly a year. In popular accounts it was
said that Major General Charles Gordon (1833-85) was killed unarmed
on the steps of the Governor-General's palace, dying passively almost as
a Christ-like figure, while around 10,000 civilians and members of the
garrison were ruthlessly massacred. The Gordon Relief Expedition (1884–
85), also known as the Nile Expedition, a mission to relieve Gordon and
the besieged garrison, began in September 1884 under the command of
General Garnet Wolseley (1833-1913). Ever since then, ETW had been
closely monitoring the expedition's progress, given that Charly had been
appointed chief of its intelligence department. By the end of December,
Charly was part of the desert column, numbering around 1,000 men
with 2,000 camels under the command of Sir Herbert Stewart (1843-85),
which was approaching Korti.[2] Then, on 18 January, Stewart was fatally
wounded, and the command devolved to Charly, despite his inexperience
of commanding troops in action.

On 7 February, for long his daily routine, ETW anxiously scanned
the newspaper columns, searching for the latest telegrams from the
Sudan. His gaze immediately fell on the headline that announced the 'Fall
of Khartoum'. The War Office telegram provided the bare facts:

> Sir Charles Wilson arrived there on the 28th to find the place in the hands
> of the enemy. He returned under heavy fire from the river banks. Steamers

in which he returned were wrecked some miles below the Shublaka Cataract. The whole party were saved, and landed on an island, where they

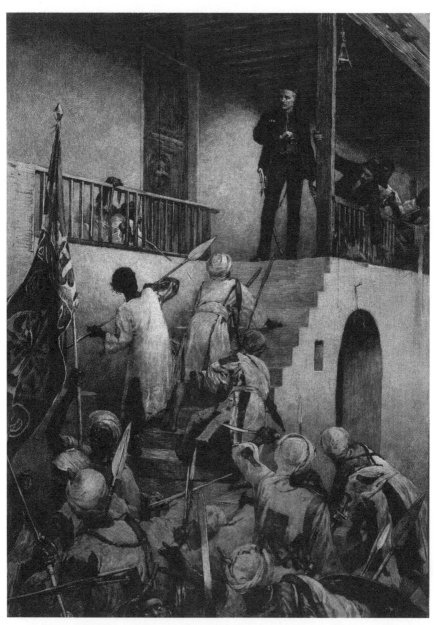

General Gordon standing on the stairs of his house about to be speared by dervishes. Etching by H. Dicksee after G. W. Joy, 1897.

are in safety. A steamer has gone to fetch them. Fate of Gordon uncertain. Lord Wolseley reports Sir H. Stewart doing well, and that nearly all the wounded were being brought to Gakdul.[3]

As he continued to read, the narrowness of Charly's escape became evident: one of his steamers had been wrecked during the journey up the Nile while the other was destroyed on the return journey. On both occasions, his men were forced to run the gauntlet of heavy fire from the armed rebels who lined the banks. The nearer they approached Khartoum, the heavier the rebel fire became, and it quickly became apparent that the palace had been overthrown by the Mahdi. Consequently, Charly had decided to turn back. At this stage, it was thought that General Gordon was being held as a hostage since the Muslims were unlikely to have killed a 'holy' man such as Gordon. Nevertheless, his death was still not being ruled out.[4]

The news of Gordon's death first broke through a despatch to the Central News Agency by the *Daily Chronicle* war correspondent Charles Frederick Williams (1838-1904). His later account, 'How we lost Gordon', published in the 1 May issue of *Fortnightly Review*, made a virulent attack on Charly. This included criticism of his perceived hesitation, unnecessary delays and failure to obtain certainty around Gordon's fate. Signed off at Korti on 9 March, six weeks after the fall of Khartoum, significantly, it was written near Wolseley's headquarters, and probably reflected Wolseley's private views and those of his closest advisers.[5]

A fortnight later, Charly was then surprised, given that he had already submitted full reports on all his actions, to be asked by Wolseley to explain why he did not depart for Khartoum before 24 January. He immediately wrote the supplementary report, which, after some delay, Wolseley forwarded to the Secretary of State for War, together with an ambiguously worded covering note[6] that could be interpreted either as praiseworthy or censorious. A bitter debate subsequently followed, played out in the full glare of the British press, in which Charly was both blamed and defended.

In the popular myth that was created in the aftermath of Gordon's death, the general became a martyred warrior-saint and his story - one which became 'known to every schoolboy'- told of British troops bravely fighting their way across the desert, only to arrive two days 'Too Late!'

However, an analysis of the campaign reveals evidence that tells a different story.[7] ETW was quick to grasp that the authorities were seeking to make Charly a scapegoat, and lay the blame of the failure to rescue Gordon on his brother's shoulders. He endeavoured to reveal the true facts, and began a campaign to defend Charly. Determining to influence public opinion as far as he could, he sent the following letter to the *Daily News*:

> Sir, - May I claim a space for a few lines in the name of fair play? Your leader on General Gordon on Tuesday last is founded entirely on an article in the *Fortnightly Review* by Mr. Chas. Williams, a gentleman whose society, as I understand, it was Sir Chas. Wilson's duty unfortunately to decline on his expedition to Khartoum. Personal feeling and pique are but too manifest throughout Mr. Williams's article; and I only ask that Sir Charles Wilson's reason should be weighed before any opinion is formed as to his "so-called" delay at Metemmeh. From a pretty good knowledge of my brother's character I feel sure that he is not the man to "lose nerve," "to hesitate," "to waste days," or "to dawdle" when work has to be done. No other act of his life shows this; and on the occasion in question his whole heart, as I know, was set upon joining hands with his friend and comrade in Khartoum. I hold therefore that your strictures are as premature as I believe them to be undeserved. - I am, yours faithfully, EDWARD T. WILSON - Cheltenham, May 6.[8]

The letter became widely disseminated, leading to the topic being discussed in all corners of the country. Perhaps this is best illustrated through the following article which appeared in the *Northern Chronicle and General Advertiser for the North of Scotland* on 27 May:

> The vigorous philippic that Mr Williams launches against Sir Charles Wilson in the current number of the *Fortnightly* has made a very palpable hit. There is nothing wonderful in that; but there is something wonderful in the fact that the retorts courteous have been at once so few and so weak. The first defence of the unfortunate officer's conduct comes from the pen of his brother, Mr Edward T. Wilson, and may be taken as a very fair illustration of zeal without knowledge. He says that "personal feeling and pique are but too manifest throughout Mr Williams' article," and that this gentleman's society "it was Sir Charles Wilson's duty, unfortunately,

to decline on his expedition to Khartoum." That may or may not be the case; but the statement, far from being an answer to the strictures of Mr Williams, only succeeds in affording a neat example of the logical fallacy known as *ignoratio elenchi*.[9]

While ETW was probably unaware of these specific remarks, his patience was undoubtedly tested with similar comments. Nevertheless, according to Charly's biographer 'the majority of the daily press took [Charly's] side in the controversy, and showed that the general feeling was entirely in favour of his action'.[10] Although there was strong local support expressed for Charly as an Old Cheltonian,[11] some quarters of the local press considered ETW's attempts 'to save his brother's reputation, though very praiseworthy, [to] be quite futile'.[12] They added:

> The edict has gone forth. It was necessary that some one should be sacrificed to defend Mr. Gladstone from the charge of procrastination, and Dr. Wilson ought to feel flattered by the selection of his brother as the victim.[13]

ETW persevered, no doubt energised by his unrelenting 'zeal' but also with his clear 'knowledge' of the facts. On 28 May, his good analytical skills came to the fore with the publication of the following letter in the *Morning Post*:

> Mr. E. T. Wilson, the brother of Sir Charles Wilson, who is likely before long to return to England from the Soudan, desires to draw attention to the fact that Sir Charles Wilson's report relative to the expedition under his command to Khartoum is dated March 23, and was in Lord Hartington's[14] hands on April 21. The article in the *Fortnightly* on the same subject was published May 1. It must be clear, therefore, he says, that his brother's report was written without any knowledge of the review article. As some misconception appears to have arisen on this point he thinks it should be corrected.[15]

Nevertheless, in the frenzied debates that followed, little effort was made in practice to establish the real facts. Right from the start, there were strong political factors at play, a fact not overlooked by the *Gloucestershire Echo*:

We are inclined to think that Dr. E. T. Wilson's opinion of the great Liberal party just at the present moment would be interesting. He does not appear to see the fun of having his brother offered up as a sort of scape-goat to bear away the sins of the Gladstone Cabinet. [...] If Sir Chas. Wilson, and not Mr. Gladstone, is morally guilty of Gordon's death, why should he escape with the punishment of his own reflections? That, to a politician, may be an appropriate punishment, but a soldier asks to be judged by a more honourable standard. Such, at least, is the view of Dr. E. T. Wilson.[16]

As things transpired, a change in government was one of the factors that proved beneficial in Charly's case. Gladstone's administration fell on 9 June and was replaced by a Conservative government led by Lord Salisbury. This eventually resulted in the release of new evidence, which ETW probably saw reported in the *Cheltenham Chronicle* on 21 July as follows:

... Viscount Bury, the new Under Secretary of State for War, has just discovered the copy of a telegram sent by the Marquis of Hartington, on February 11th, 1885, to General Wolseley, in the following terms: *"Express warm recognition of Government of brilliant services of Sir Charles Wilson, and satisfaction at gallant rescue of his party."* When the Parliamentary papers upon the subject were issued by the late Ministry, this telegram was not included, and would never have seen the light of day but for the change of Government. The only explanation offered is that "by some means" the telegram was "accidentally omitted." Accidents we know *will* happen, but it is rather suggestive that, whilst this particular telegram was being "accidentally" suppressed by the Ministry, the recognised organ of the Liberal party was defending the Government from the responsibility of the fall of Khartoum, by attributing the disaster to the cowardice and inaction of Sir Charles Wilson.[17]

The following year, Charly published a more detailed account entitled *From Korti to Khartum* (1886) to further support his version of the facts.[18] It was also covered in his biography, published by his friend Sir Charles Watson (1844-1916) in 1909.[19] Watson commented:

The book ... was received enthusiastically both by Wilson's friends and by the press, as it was universally regarded as a full and complete answer to the charge of delay which had been brought against him, in order to screen others from the blame due to them for the failure of the Nile expedition.[20]

While Charly's name was fully cleared, and he was even created a KCB for his service in the Sudan, ETW continued to feel how pitiful it was 'that so many years should have been clouded by malicious slander and undeserved neglect by those who were themselves to blame ...'.[21] It was a far cry from when the two brothers were innocently bathing, fishing, and rowing along the Pembrokeshire coast, or playing imaginary smuggling games in the caves. There, they had avoided getting caught up in the neighbouring quicksand; but, at that time, they could never have predicted other forms of 'quicksand' that might, one day, stand in their way. Thankfully, the 'Fall of Khartoum' was one which, though painful and treacherous, did not succeed in swallowing them up.

12
Country Living (1885–6)

Medical Officer of Health – *The Crippetts* – Mind reading – Hospital
politics – Pleuropneumonia

*'... many was the nightmare that I had during the first winter when everything
had to be bought and carted up the hill from the town'.*
~ ETW ~

D URING FEBRUARY 1885, AS ETW eagerly scanned the papers for
news of Charly's fate in the Sudan, he also anxiously awaited news
of his application for the post of Medical Officer of Health. As early as
1867 he had advocated the need for such a position,[1] despite facing
strong political objections, namely: that if a town was so unhealthy as to
need a Medical Officer of Health,[2] then it could never be frequented as
a watering place. Now, following the death of Dr Thomas Wright (1809-
84) on 17 November, the position had become vacant. ETW had been
strongly encouraged to apply and, if successful, intended to continue to
practise as a consulting physician. His election was considered a practical
certainty, the *Cheltenham Examiner* setting out his excellent credentials
and undoubted popularity should he be chosen. It commented:

> Dr. WILSON's knowledge of the sanitary condition of the town, and
> especially of the incidence of its water supply, is second to that of no man,
> now that his old friend and fellow-worker, Dr. WRIGHT, has been removed.
> It is a knowledge acquired by many years of study and experience. Before
> the office of Medical Officer of Health was established, and when sanitary
> science was not the fashionable pursuit it is now, Dr. WILSON did useful
> service in directing attention to the wants of some of the worst districts
> of the town; and the paper read by him, just twenty years ago, before the
> British Association at Bath, on "Sanitary Statistics of Cheltenham," was a
> remarkable proof of the mass of information he had even then acquired.
> Dr. WILSON's election would undoubtedly be a popular one, and it is no

disparagement of other claims to the vacant office to say that it would be difficult to find one who would discharge its duties with equal abillty.[3]

Nevertheless, it was not to be. A genial Irish surgeon, Dr Roche, was appointed. While he was the only one in the pool of thirty-five candidates who lacked suitable qualifications, significantly, Roche was first cousin of the senior official responsible for managing the role. As ETW remarked, '[Dr Roche] was as much surprised as anyone to find himself successful, [and] rushed off to make good his deficiency at the University of Dublin'.[4] Following this shameless case of nepotism, '[ETW's] faith in Town Councils was shaken forever after'.[5]

~~~

I N SEPTEMBER, THE FAMILY decided not to renew the lease on the farm at *Sunnymede*. Instead, they leased a new farm, *The Crippetts*, which was situated about three miles outside Cheltenham. The farm was balanced on the edge of the Cotswolds on a long spur of Leckhampton Hill, near the village of Shurdington. The unusual name of 'Crippetts' is thought to derive from 'Cropet' or 'Crupet', a common Middle-English surname in Gloucestershire during the thirteenth century. Originally, *The Crippetts* consisted of a single two-storey cottage with farm buildings. Today,

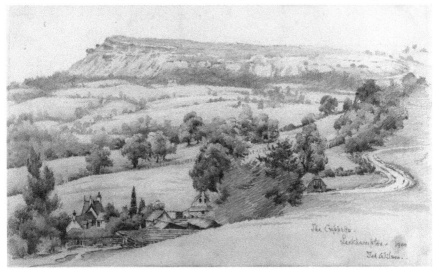

The Crippetts. 1900. Drawing by Ted Wilson.

although it has been divided into private dwellings, it still retains much of its original character, the cottage still maintaining the black and white timbered façade.[6] The Tudor farm cottage stood on a site that had been occupied and farmed for many hundreds of years, at this time employing in the region of ten people, although the Bailiff was soon replaced due to his drunken inclinations. The lease was no light undertaking, costing £230 per year (equivalent to £16,000 today). The logistics of fitting out the farm with the right equipment and furnishings were also not straightforward and exercised ETW's organisational abilities during the first winter. Here, Mary could indulge her new interest in Dexter Cattle. While she achieved early success with rearing boar, winning first prize (£5) at the 1887 annual meeting of the Gloucestershire Agricultural Society,[7] and producing milk from Alderney and Shorthorn Cattle,[8] the venture with Dexter Cattle subsequently proved unsuccessful after the animals became overfed.[9]

This unspoilt corner of the Cotswolds provided excellent opportunities, particularly for ETW and Ted, to explore the natural world on their doorstep. The woods, fields and hedgerows were teeming with wildlife of every sort: badgers and foxes, red squirrels and rabbits, grass snakes, newts, birds and insects in profusion. Particular comment was made on the wonderful number of butterflies which abounded on the estate. ETW was gratified that Ted and Bernard would be able to 'get into country habits',[10] riding, shooting and dabbling in estate management. Later, Bernard went on to become a recognised dowser. ETW also commented that his daughters had benefitted too from 'the open air life and surroundings'.[11] Many of the following summer holidays were spent by the entire family at *The Crippetts* where they enjoyed 'the fine bracing air and thorough country life'.[12]

While *The Crippetts* became the family's escape from everyday pressures, for a while *Westal* became a place where experiments in mind reading took place. Perhaps influenced by ETW's recent paper[13] on 'The Mind's Eye', read before the Cheltenham Natural Science Society (CNSS), Mary participated in some novel experiments: according to the Society for Psychical Research she used her will, with apparent success, to influence the physical actions of an acquaintance.[14] ETW kept an open mind on mental phenomena such as hypnotism and telepathy.[15] Based on his experience with unusual hospital cases he recognised how the eye's vision could be deceived through 'the sensory ganglia in the brain – the mind's eye – where the impression becomes a sensation, and gives rise to ideas, to emotions, or the higher intellectual operations'.[16] In this way, a blind patient of his was able to see flashes of light which resembled gas flames. He concluded:

> In each case the consciousness is deceived, and confounds an impression caused by injury of the sensory nerve itself, with an impression coming through the ordinary channel of the external sense organ, be this the eye, or the ear, or the nose, or the organ of common sense.[17]

A little later, he presented another paper to the CNSS, this time on 'The nerve mechanisms of articulate speech'. He wrote:

> That we should have two minds acting independently but in focus, as it were, without knowing it, is no more wonderful than that we should see with two eyes at once, or with one only, and be unable to say which eye is acting. On the face of it, it seems possible, if not probable, that the two hemispheres [of the brain] may act separately but in harmony, and, if so, it is not surprising if, under certain conditions, they may act inharmoniously as a mental squint, and give rise to some of the mental phases which have been a puzzle to psychologists.[18]

In an age of new scientific discovery, ETW was excited to consider that 'The unknown, in all probability, exceeds the known, … and Science has as many triumphs before her in the future as she can boast in the past'.[19] While he did not dismiss Mary's experiments as being of no scientific value, he was quick to distinguish truth from deception. A few years earlier, at a thought reading party at a fellow doctor's house, which he and Mary attended, he recorded that the doctor's daughter 'did some very clever tricks'.[20] Later, replicating these at home, he commented:

> It was not 'Thought reading' but muscle reading for resistance was at once felt in the hand covering the eyes when the marked object was quickly passed.[21]

~~~

D URING FEBRUARY 1886, A year after ETW's unsuccessful bid to become Cheltenham's second Medical Officer of Health, mismanagement once again surfaced. This time, the controversy concerned the election of a new Surgeon at the General Hospital.[22] In another clear case of 'cliquey management'[23] the leading candidate, G. Arthur Cardew, was rejected unfairly; ETW opined that he 'had unfortunately to bear the (supposed) sins of his father who had been Chaplain to the Hospital …'.[24] While ETW did his best to challenge the decision,[25] it was to no avail; the repercussions were far-reaching and led to much boardroom in-fighting, an inquiry, and a report which, ETW thought, 'put the clock back at the Hospital for some years …'.[26] ETW's displeasure about the handling of hospital affairs was soon forgotten, however, when, during the spring, his practice became inundated with cases arising from a severe epidemic of pleuropneumonia. In one Ladies' College Boarding House alone, he had five cases of empyema (the presence of pus in the pleural space) requiring operation. In another two cases, both patients died, one after requiring surgery to remove six ribs.[27] By August, he was relieved to spend restorative moments with the family at *The Crippetts*; here, he regained some strength before embarking on further projects.

13
Salubritas et Eruditio (1886-93)

Revival of Cheltenham Spa – Montpellier Gardens – Victoria Nursing
Home – Royal Crescent Library – School of Art –'The water we drink' –
Delancey management issues – CNSS Presidency – Family celebrations
and misfortunes – Offer of mayorship

*'My object in bringing the subject forward is to draw out your sympathy – if
possible your enthusiasm – in the revival of our Cheltenham Spa'.*
~ ETW ~

EVER SINCE THE 1830S, there had been a gradual decline in the
fashion of drinking water at British inland resorts. This was fuelled
partly by the popularity of seaside holidays in the UK and, following the
establishment of peace in Europe after the end of the Napoleonic Wars
(1803-15), the attraction of foreign spas. Once hailed as the 'Queen of
English Watering Places' Cheltenham had drastically scaled down its
facilities as a spa. As ETW observed in a letter to the *Cheltenham Examiner*
in January 1886, the town focused on 'catering only for winter visitors to
the neglect of those who might come in the summer season and drink her
waters as of old'.[1] In contrast, he highlighted how Bath and Leamington
had recently improved their infrastructure as spas, and bemoaned the
following:

> Cheltenham possesses no public garden or place of resort where a visitor
> could sit or walk without paying for the privilege; its baths are quite
> unworthy of the town; and the mineral waters, which are as efficacious
> now as they ever were, are either disused or offered for sale to the highest
> bidder.[2]

Five years earlier, in December 1880, he had welcomed the French
physician Henri Cazalis (1840-1909), then acting as medical consultant at
Aix-les-Bains, to accompany him on a tour of the town's spas and walks.
On that occasion, the two doctors shared their disbelief concerning the

town authorities' indifference towards the development of the spas.[3] Nevertheless, in 1887, when Cheltenham officially received its arms and a crest, it chose *Salubritas et Eruditio* (meaning 'Through Health and Learning') as its motto. With *Salubritas* celebrating its heritage as a spa and Eruditio its reputation as an important educational centre, perhaps this was to signal a new golden age in the town's fortunes.

In March 1886, when various ideas were put forward to celebrate Queen Victoria's Golden Jubilee, including the provision of a public library, the purchase of the Marle Hill Estate to convert it into a public park, and the acquisition of the Winter Garden, ETW proposed the purchase of Montpellier Gardens. Originally laid out in 1831, the Gardens were conceived as exclusive pleasure grounds for visitors to Montpellier Spa. Rather than converting them into a people's park, ETW's concern was 'chiefly for the visitors who were coming to the town to take the waters'.[4] He thought that by presenting them to the town through a scheme costing £8,500 they would revive the summer season in Cheltenham, traditionally considered the best time for taking its waters. Having previously contributed to a pamphlet[5] promoting the benefits and methods of taking the mineral waters at Montpellier Spa, this was a subject close to his heart.

While his project was not selected as the preferred Jubilee scheme, ETW helped to ensure, through his chairmanship of the relevant committee, that in 1897 the Town Council purchased Montpellier Gardens, together with Montpellier Baths and the rights to the many mineral wells in the town. In 1892, in a series of letters published in the *Cheltenham Examiner*,[6] he also stimulated a public debate about the revival of the town's spas. Drawing on research in the *British Medical Journal* he suggested that the German town of Carlsbad (now Karlovy Vary in the Czech Republic) could be used as a blueprint for Cheltenham's development. Noting that its waters still presented Carlsbad's principal attraction, he recognised that they formed only part of a combined cure - catering for both mind and body - consisting of air, music, and exercise. If Cheltenham could emulate Carlsbad, a town with a population of just 12,000, ETW was sure it could eventually rank among Europe's elite watering places and, like Carlsbad, attract 30,000 visitors annually.

As part of a strategy for realising the vision, ETW suggested that chemical analyses of the waters should be conducted and their healing powers re-assessed against the latest and more stringent standards governing the use of modern medication. Having already consulted Dr Hermann Weber (1823-1918),[7] one of Europe's authorities on mineral waters, he was optimistic that this approach would yield success. In future, he thought, local doctors would prescribe waters for a range of illnesses, including gout, anaemia and diseases of the kidney and liver. Additionally, ETW's plan envisaged the Town Council acquiring ownership of the mineral wells; conducting a survey to re-discover springs previously lost or built over; and replacing obsolete pumping equipment.

To cater for exercise and fresh air, ETW recommended that beauty spots such as Leckhampton Hill could be made more accessible via a 'toy train' or charabanc service. The Carlsbad model, he suggested, could also be copied through engaging bands for the 'music cure'; promoting the town's existing baths (both ordinary and medicinal) for relaxation and health; and even encouraging local bakers to produce high quality bread and coffee for a diet of continental breakfasts. While investment costs would be high, these could be offset through cure and music taxes, which brought in an annual income of £25,000 in Carlsbad; and additional revenue could be gained through the sale of different types of Cheltenham salts and bottled waters.

Having formulated his preliminary ideas and gained initial interest in the scheme from the majority of Town Councillors, ETW then presented them for critical scrutiny to the Cheltenham Debating Society.[8] 'Everything will depend', he cautioned, 'upon the way in which the thing is done'.[9] Therefore, he encouraged other ideas and models to be suggested and examined before deciding on a final approach. While ETW favoured Carlsbad and other French and German spas as possible models, he recommended not imitating them slavishly:

> Whatever we do, let us be distinctive: taking hints everywhere, adopting the good and discarding the bad ....[10]

He also shared a vision for a new Central Spa, which he described as 'a grand and lofty hall ... adapted to many uses, water drinking, musical promenades, possibly lectures and balls',[11] next to which, given the vagaries of the local climate, would stand a glass house used for exercising in bad weather. Nevertheless, while his ideas received much approval, they failed to secure convincing widespread support. Despite this, he continued to champion the cause. During August, for example, while on a fishing trip in Yorkshire, he visited Harrogate, a town still flourishing as a spa. Spurred on by a local guide-book, claiming that to travel from Cheltenham or Bath to Harrogate was like 'a transition from death to life – from the past to the present',[12] ETW went to investigate for himself. Here, he found a 'thoroughly go ahead English spa',[13] where there was as much vibrancy at 7.30 in the morning as Cheltenham only experienced at 4 o'clock in the afternoon on a fine spring or autumn day. Moreover, he discovered, Harrogate's population more than trebled through its influx of annual visitors who enjoyed state-of-the-art leisure and exercise facilities. Writing up his experience in two *Cheltenham Examiner* articles,[14] he concluded:

> The raw material lies around us in ample profusion, if we only know how to use it, and nothing seems wanting for success if we have but faith in ourselves, a well-defined goal, and a fixed resolve that no stone shall be left unturned to reach it.[15]

Nevertheless, repeated attempts to revive the spa, including proposals to erect a Kursaal and baths at the south end of the Winter Garden, ended in failure.[16] ETW was particularly annoyed when the scheme became identified with a certain Town Councillor, that of Dr G. H. Ward-Humphreys.[17] Previously, the two doctors had crossed swords when Ward-Humphreys promoted water from the River Severn as being safe to drink. Further scope for conflict arose following Ward-Humphreys' appointment as Hon. Sec. of the Medical Spa Committee in 1893. The latter's reputation of exercising a 'masterful personality' and having a great 'hold upon the popular imagination' (once being taunted in a Town Council meeting for 'being able to hypnotise any representative committee')[18] probably did not endear him to ETW. Preferring a less bombastic approach, ETW would have shuddered at the councillor's 'active and versatile temperament' and the resulting columns in the local press which 'were filled with controversy concerning his objects and methods'.[19]

~~~

ALTHOUGH ETW'S SUGGESTION FOR Montpellier Gardens was not selected as a Jubilee scheme, another project that he supported was. In May 1887, under the aegis of the Nursing Branch of the Charity Organisation Society, which he helped to establish in 1879, he led an appeal to purchase a home for six district nurses and a Lady Superintendent. While the existing staff comprised two trained nurses and a midwife, an extra two nurses and another midwife, assisted where necessary by untrained nurses, were considered necessary to provide efficient nursing for the whole town.[20] By October, good progress had been achieved and, at an important meeting at the Assembly Rooms, ETW reported that funding of £1,000 had been secured. During spring 1888, the building, known as the Victoria Home, was opened in St George's Place. Three years later, it moved to larger premises in St James's Square, opposite the Great Western Railway station, accommodating additional staff and incorporating a small ward for maternity patients.[21] Then, in 1896, as chairman of the District Nursing Association's Executive Committee, ETW appealed for further funding to develop the Home. At a meeting in the Imperial Rooms he canvassed for new subscribers by outlining the considerable improvements which the nurses had brought. By focusing care on 'the aged, helpless and hopelessly ill' they had filled a vital gap for patients who were unable to be admitted either to the General Hospital or the Delancey. Care had also been provided to some complex cases, including eighteen paralytics and thirty-two patients suffering from cancer, heart disease, and consumption. In ETW's view they brought 'order out of chaos' and 'comfort and care and cleanliness' wherever they went.[22]

Final success was achieved at a large meeting at the Winter Garden in March 1897 when a resolution to use the Queen Victoria's Diamond Jubilee Memorial Fund to support the development of the Victoria Nursing Home was seconded by ETW. Describing how the demand for its services, now in its seventeenth year, had increased, he reported proudly that the staff (comprising a matron and eight nurses, including two maternity nurses) had made 17,000 visits during 1896 and attended nearly 300 maternity cases.[23] Later, in 1904, when the Cheltenham District Nursing Association celebrated its silver jubilee, ETW was able to report on the

Home's further success: in just one year, the nurses attended 1,442 cases in the town and made 37,947 visits.[24]

~~~

APART FROM FOCUSING ON initiatives related to *Salubritas* ETW also supported *Eruditio* in several ways, including as a member of the Ladies' College Council and as Secretary, and, later, President, of the Royal Crescent Library. Established in 1863, this private subscription library was located at 5 Royal Crescent. Prior to the establishment of a free library in 1884, another cause vigorously supported by ETW, it contained the town's most significant collection of books and journals.[25] By 1901, however, the Crescent Library started to diminish in importance. Noting the establishment of rival libraries, particularly at Cheltenham College and the Ladies' College, ETW commented: 'Few books of worth are read and novels are required in ever increasing numbers'.[26] When the library closed in 1908,[27] however, it was ETW who ensured that its collection was safely transferred to the public library.

Another educational institution, which he vigorously supported, was the Cheltenham School of Art.[28] As its secretary during a critical period of its development he oversaw the public appeal to raise funds for its new building. Founded in 1852 the Cheltenham School was among the earliest in the country, but its premises, located then in Clarence Parade, had fallen into disrepair. Faulty lighting and inadequate accommodation were causing difficulties, while average class numbers had trebled to thirty within two years from 1881. Moreover, the number of works submitted to the National Art Training School (now part of the Royal College of Art) at South Kensington, London had increased from 450 to 750 in just one year.[29] Given that schools of art relied on subscriptions in aid as well as fees from students and government grants, ETW drew attention to the mismatch in funding in Cheltenham's case. While Belfast contributed £761 annually to its School, and Newport £162, a wealthy and cultured town like Cheltenham only contributed occasional donations of prizes for local competitions. In his view it was not a case of supporting 'Art for art's sake'; rather, when viewed from the socio-economic point of view, it was about 'developing the talent latent among English workmen and workwomen ... and enabling them to hold ground hitherto almost abandoned to those trained in foreign studios'.[30] Support for this was then achieved in 1887 when ETW happily announced that the school would now be housed in the new public library building in Clarence Street.[31]

Around two years later, on 20 May 1889, it was officially opened to the public in its new premises.[32] The distinguished artist William Yeames (1835-1918), one of Mary's relatives, gave the address. While there were grounds for optimism about the school's future, following the successful appeal to the public, there was still doubt about its long-term funding. The Town Council had not stepped forward to offer a subscription in aid and, with the National Art Training School deciding not to contribute emergency lifeline income, ETW and the fundraising committee turned to local patrons to provide the necessary shortfall in the interim. Eventually, the school became amalgamated with Cheltenham Grammar School, and ETW continued his support for it through joining the school's governing body.

~~~

I N ADDITION TO THIS *Eruditio* issue, one *Salubritas* matter that arose during this period related to the town's water supply. This was partly prompted by ETW who, in October 1888, achieved his desire to make water supply one of the key issues at local government elections. Though not naming him directly, ETW wrote a letter to the local press criticising William Hands, the Liberal candidate for the North Ward, for the following:

> ... being an advocate of sewage drink for his neighbours, and with being an opponent of the introduction of anything in purer form as an interference with the liberty of the subject.[33]

Inevitably, it sparked an angry response. Hands demanded ETW to withdraw his assertion, but ETW remained steadfast, maintaining his position that he would only vote for a candidate who would improve the town's sanitation and ensure a free supply of pure water for the poor, who still drank from polluted wells.

ETW raised further issues the following April when he presented a paper at the Cheltenham Natural Science Society. Entitled 'The water we drink' the paper drew attention to the slow progress being made by the

Town Council to increase the number of houses supplied with hill water. The process was slow and tedious: legally, a well could not be compulsorily closed until there was undisputed proof that it was polluted, and additional resistance arose from ignorant tenants and greedy landlords.[34] Inevitably, ETW warned, this would result in repeated outbreaks of typhoid emanating from polluted shallow wells on the sand bed. Earlier, he questioned:

> Are we to sit complacently by with brimming reservoirs and storage sufficient for the best part of a twelvemonth, and for the sake of a few paltry pence in the shape of water rates, allow the poor to sicken and die for the lack of wholesome drink? Shall we subscribe to Coffee Taverns, Teetotal Societies, and the like, and leave these poor people with water which we should ourselves turn from with disgust and dismay? [35]

Given that the current policy was costing the town more in terms of economic loss and reputational impact through the spread of infectious diseases than the loss of thousands of gallons of water, he argued that Cheltenham - as a fashionable watering place and centre of education - could ill afford another typhoid epidemic. Putting it bluntly, he suggested:

> No mercy should be shown to grasping landlords who deny to their tenants this first necessity of existence. At the same time no petty difficulties should be placed in the way of those who are inclined to do their duty. The poor should not be subjected to inconveniences which the rich would not tolerate. Above all, there should be a set determination that at whatever cost the poor people on the sandbed should be supplied with a boon which they would soon learn to estimate at its true value.[36]

Nevertheless, ETW's pleas largely fell on deaf ears. Although it was nearly thirty years since he first became embroiled in the quest for clean drinking water, it would still remain an unresolved issue well into the next century. Similar levels of perseverance were also required to deal with various management issues affecting the Delancey Hospital. During this period, it was the increasingly strained relations between the latter and the General Hospital that occupied much of ETW's mind. Initially, a dispute broke out in February 1888 between the General Hospital Board and the Delancey Hospital Trustees. As ETW put it, the Board was intent on 'ungenerously demanding their pound of flesh in the form of admission of their diphtheria cases'.[37] The expectation was that they would be treated free of charge in the Delancey despite there being no special provision to cater for diphtheria. Although the Delancey agreed to do this, no cases transpired. Nevertheless, it underlined the importance of accelerating construction of the Delancey's new Diphtheria Block. While diphtheria presented no immediate threats, during the autumn a severe typhoid epidemic struck the town. The wards at the General Hospital were soon overwhelmed by the volume of cases, causing the Delancey to accommodate some. Despite this, ETW cautiously strove to ensure that the hospital maintained its independence. In June 1889, he strongly opposed the Cheltenham Improvement Act as this included a clause allowing the Town Council to share in the management of the hospital. However, by 1893 agreement was reached to allow this to happen in consideration of an annual subsidy.

~~~

WHILE MANAGERIAL CHALLENGES SOMETIMES sapped ETW's energy, he was able to find positive stimulation through other pursuits. On 3 October 1889, for example, he was elected as President of the CNSS,[38] a position he was to hold for twenty-five years. One of his first tasks was to introduce a lecture at the Assembly Rooms by the Revd Dr William Dallinger (1839-1909), a former President of the Royal Microscopical Society. It fitted well with the society's aim: 'to diffuse a love of science by monthly meetings, at which papers ... on scientific subjects were read, and followed by discussion'.[39] It also appealed to ETW's interest in photomicrography. Entitled 'Contrasts in Nature: the infinitely great and the infinitely small', Dallinger's talk charmed his audience by exposing them to the exciting new opportunities provided by the telescope and microscope. It included a series of photomicrographs on lantern slides to reveal the intricacies of chalk as an example of organic rock and showed in extraordinary detail how the chalk foraminifera (single-celled organisms) adjusted to diverse surroundings. Dallinger also displayed desmids (a division of green algae), whose three dimensions in total measured less than sixty-millionths of an inch, providing yet another example of 'the infinite mystery of life'.[40]

While the talk by Dallinger enthralled ETW, one given by the controversial missionary and nurse, Kate Marsden (1859-1931) a few years later, on 24 February 1893, achieved the opposite outcome. Recounting her alleged work on leprosy in Siberia, published as *On Sledge and Horseback to Outcast Siberian Lepers* (1893), ETW heard Marsden describe how her party was forced 'to encounter terrible snow storms, to wade through marshes, to penetrate forests of burning peat, and to cross dangerous rivers'.[41] Aware that the veracity of her journey was being called into question in some quarters, ETW asked her afterwards 'if she had ever fallen in with an elk in the wilds'.[42] When she replied by asking 'What is an elk?', he concluded that she had not travelled through Siberia at all and was, in his opinion, an 'arch humbug'.[43]

~~~

DURING THIS PERIOD, MUCH of Wilson family life was marked by celebration. On 21 June 1887, the day of celebration for Queen Victoria's Golden Jubilee, the entire family went to *The Crippetts* to watch the lighting of the celebratory beacons. In the perfectly clear conditions, they spotted a remarkable ninety bonfires along the length of the Severn Valley, from Leckhampton Hill to the Wrekin, ETW recalling the following lines from Lord Macaulay's famous poem 'The Armada' (1832):

Till twelve fair counties saw the blaze on Malvern's lonely height,
Till streamed in crimson on the wind the Wrekin's crest of light.

Later, in July 1889, further celebration occurred with the arrival of another daughter, the final expansion of the Wilson family. Gwladys Elizabeth took the total number of children to ten, although following the early death of Jessie, it was never higher than nine at any one time. Gwladys became a firm favourite with the whole family but particularly with ETW. 'It was a renewal of a life', he commented, 'which shed nothing but joy and gladness ...'.[44] Tragically, in August 1894, shortly after the family was helping with the hay making at *The Crippetts*,[45] Gwladys died suddenly of an unknown fever. For ETW, so often the curer of fevers, this was especially hard to bear.[46] Ted and his brothers, with staff from *The Crippetts*, carried her to her resting place at Leckhampton, where many

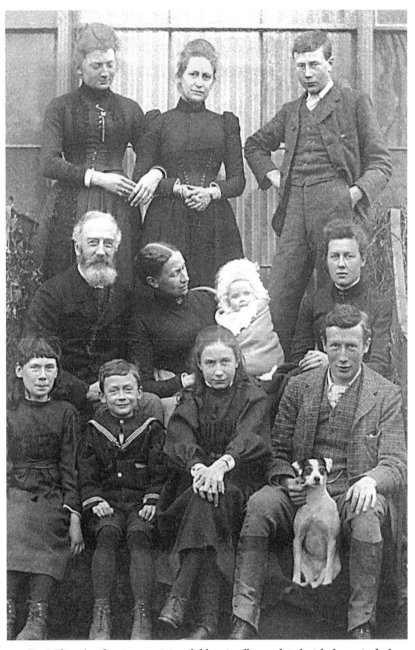

The Wilson family, nine surviving children in all, completed with the arrival of Gwladys in 1889. L-R: Back Row: Pollie; Lilly; Ted; Middle Row: ETW; Mary with Gwladys; Nellie; Front Row: Elsie; Jim; Ida; Bernard (with Minnie).

of the family were eventually to lie. The family then repaired to Nevin, in North Wales for a holiday to come to terms with their loss.

Several of the children were now spreading their wings and leaving home. In 1889, Bernard gained a diploma from the Royal Agricultural College in Cirencester, and went to Yorkshire where he became a land agent. In 1891, Nellie was in South Africa, training to be a nurse, while Ted went up to Gonville and Caius College, Cambridge to study Natural Science. Earlier, ETW's poem, following the usual family tradition of penning some doggerel verse to accompany each Christmas gift, seemed quite revealing as regards his thoughts on Ted's future career path:

A box full of curios, here, I bring
For Master Teddie's Christmasing
Skull of Turtle – skull of Dog
Skull of a huge Hedgehog;
Of money too I heard the clink
It might have been the missing link
That leads from Monkey to the Man
If we believe in Darwin's plan.
Soon you'll be licensed, Sir, to kill
Man, woman, child who's maimed or ill
Be sure you use your license kindly
Don't cut or even phisick blindly
Prepare your pills with brains and then
You'll cure not kill your fellow men.[47]

Fervent celebration also occurred following Charly's appointment as Director-General of the Ordnance Survey (OS), in Southampton. During a visit there in August 1889, ETW met one of General Gordon's sisters who showed him the original manuscripts of Gordon's journal which she donated to the OS collections. Nine months later, on 24 May 1890, ETW attended the formal opening of a Home[48] for the Gordon Boys' Brigade in Cheltenham.[49] Primarily founded by Charly[50] in memory of General Gordon, the organisation was taken up in several towns and cities with 'the object of providing employment for destitute boys, of assisting them to obtain situations, and helping those, who were suitable, to emigrate'.[51]

~~~

S ADLY, THE PERIOD WAS also marked by misfortune. Before Bernard left Cheltenham, he suffered a serious accident at *The Crippetts* when his 'run away' horse nearly collided with the iron railings at the top of the hill. Although he managed to avoid crashing into the railings, he was knocked unconscious for fifteen hours after hitting an ash tree. For a year or more, he suffered from headaches, but, thereafter, made a good recovery. A few weeks later, in 1890, it was ETW's turn to suffer a near-fatal experience. While out shooting on a steep bank, he slipped, then fell on some pointed stakes left after a bush was cut. Had it not been for a rib, which broke after saving his fall, it could have been far more serious, especially if the pleura had been pierced. A few years later, there was further misfortune when a large fire at *Westal* shortly before Christmas of 1893 caused the usual jollity of the occasion to be rather muted. The situation was made worse by the insurance investigator whom ETW described as an 'odious, offensive little toad who seemed to think we had set things on fire on purpose'.[52] Of particular annoyance to ETW were the books in his study; these became more damaged through water than fire after the firemen overzealously doused everything. Nevertheless, it could have been far worse had a policeman not discovered the fire, by chance, whilst on his beat.[53]

Out of all the incidents that occurred to ETW during this time, there is perhaps one that sums up the considerable esteem in which he was held. On 16 December 1891, a date which happened to coincide with his fifty-ninth birthday, ETW was approached about becoming an alderman so that, the following year, he could be offered the mayorship of Cheltenham. Although he was offered financial assistance, nevertheless, he declined. 'My talents, whatever they be', he commented, 'certainly do not lie in the direction of Municipal Government'.[54] Despite this, there were few fellow citizens who expended as much energy as he on promoting the twin elements encapsulated in the town's motto – *Salubritas et Eruditio*.

14
The Conservationist (1894-6)

'Man and the Extinction of Species' – Morality of field sports –
Birdnesting

*'After stripping the Atlantic coast, the plume hunters are now at work on the
shores of Mexico, in Central America, and on the Amazon, and alas that it
should be so, the ladies of England are still the chief patrons of the cruel and
inhuman trade'.*
~ ETW ~

WHEN ETW GAVE HIS presidential address to inaugurate the 1894-5 session of the Cheltenham Natural Science Society, he chose a topic that had been exercising his mind for some time – that of human beings' ability to destroy the natural world. Earlier, his interest in wildlife conservation had largely manifested itself through papers presented to the Friends in Council between 1869 and 1871. One of these covered Charles Waterton (1782-1865), the naturalist who famously enclosed his Yorkshire estate with a 9 feet-high wall to turn it into the world's first wildlife sanctuary. Now, his new paper entitled 'Man and the Extinction of Species'[1] focused on the global destruction that only those with a detailed knowledge of the problem could fully understand.

The facts he presented spoke for themselves. Within the UK, the avocet, bustard and godwit had stopped breeding in Norfolk following the practice of draining the broads between 1825 and 1855; and in 1893 not a single great skua chick was raised on the island of Foula, in the Shetlands, after two sloops stopped to collect dozens of eggs from their nests. In the USA, the evidence was particularly damning in the case of the American Bison whose numbers had fallen by 1.5 million from 1872 to 1874. 'It is a melancholy instance of what man can do in a very few years', ETW commented, 'under the influence of greed combined with an instinct for the chase'.[2] The greed was not restricted to the land: in the oceans, whales were becoming rarer because of the industry, which sold whalebone for £1,300 (£2,650 when supply was low) per ton. Herds of buffalo had also been wiped out in Uganda because of the accidental introduction of anthrax, spread by humans. Equally devastating was the impact of the trade in fur and feathers. ETW commented:

> The demand ... is increasing – of furs for my lady in her carriage and for the Jehu on the box: of feathers for the hats and bonnets, and ball dresses of young English girls whose hearts would be touched at the death of a pigeon, but are apparently callous to the hecatomb of bright-plumaged birds slain yearly during the breeding season for their use, and the demand creates the hunter, reckless and wantonly wasteful in the pursuit of game.[3]

It was clear to ETW that the scale of destruction was accelerating at an unparalleled rate. While the introduction of firearms had given human beings, originally just primitive hunters, the upper hand over the animal kingdom, greater impact was now being caused through the practices of tilling the soil, cultivating crops, clearing forests, draining marshes and ploughing prairies. These altered and led to the loss of habitat. Moreover, severe destruction was being caused by hunting. He noted:

> Against the professional hunter of the present day on horseback, armed with the modern rifle and the explosive bullet, no game has a chance. He kills everything, bulls, cows, and half-grown calves. So that unless some stringent measures are taken to prevent it, many of the largest and the most beautiful and the most useful of existing mammalia must speedily disappear.[4]

As a hunter himself, ETW questioned the morality of field sports.[5] In his autobiographical notes, he recalled how the gun had given him 'an infinite source of pleasure'.[6] His passion for shooting began when his father gave him a small single-barrelled gun at the age of eight, which he used to kill his first bird, a robin, and his enjoyment continued well into old age. However, while enjoying hunting as a pastime, he also promoted conservation and restraint, especially when rare or endangered species were concerned. He commented:

> It is not every sportsman who knows when to stay his hand and cry "Hold, enough." Nor are all sportsmen embued with the Naturalist which is such

a welcome and redeeming feature when it peeps out in a book devoted to slaughter.[7]

The book to which ETW referred was *Big Game Shooting* (1894). From this, he quoted an incident when the big game hunter and collector Clement St George Royds Littledale (1851–1931) was tempted to shoot a magnificent bull aurochs but decided not to 'out of respect for a noble representative of a nearly extinct species'.[8] While ETW agreed with Littledale that the hunter had a moral responsibility to avoid exterminating rare species for mere wanton sport, he was also adamant that positive action should be taken to counter the human race's so-called 'right to destroy the lower order of creation for his own purposes', whether for food, clothing, decoration or sport.[9] Therefore, he advocated the passing of laws to protect the most useful and attractive creatures, and also provided support for societies such as the Selborne Society[10] which, at that time, was campaigning against the trade in bird's feathers for use in fashion. It was horrifying to discover that as much as 172,000 lbs. of feathers were imported into the country in just one year. ETW also pointed to the need for education, not only to dispel common myths held by gamekeepers, farmers, and gardeners on the necessity to destroy wildlife, but also to teach in schools 'a love for the *living* creatures and a study of life in place of skins and skeletons ...'.[11]; and he stressed the importance of recording - through photographs, drawings and accurate scientific measurements of skins and skeletons – any species that were likely to disappear. He warned:

> Much that is beautiful, much that is useful, must inevitably pass away for ever. From circumstances beyond his control man is destined before many centuries have elapsed to crowd out and destroy most of the surviving links in the chain of evolution.[12]

Two years later, ETW once again returned to the subject of conservation. In October 1896, he spoke on 'Birdnesting' for his CNSS presidential address. As one of his favourite pursuits he recognised that it received a bad reputation. On the contrary, however, he sought to show how, if carried out humanely and scientifically, it could provide 'the best means for becoming acquainted with [birds'] appearance, habits and peculiarities'.[13] To illustrate what to avoid, he shared the following story from his own experience:

> Stealing quietly through some orchards, observing my friends the warblers, a confused hubbub of voices struck my ear, and soon after, three or four schoolboys, I am not going to name the school, came along, 'eyes in air and talking loudly, on the look out for nests. Presently the nest of a chaffinch was spied, neatly-concealed on the lichen-covered branch of a pear tree. There was great rejoicing, especially when the first boy to climb up cried out that the bird was still there. Such close sitting should have told them that the eggs were useless, but this lesson had not been learned, or was forgotten in the excitement of the moment, and five hard eggs were speedily stowed away, the nest torn down in very wantonness, and the boys went on their way.[14]

By sharing this cautionary tale ETW hoped to promote the idea that boys' hunting instinct could be subdued and channelled towards the instinct of a true naturalist. In this way, he thought, 'the ruthless collector may become the most ardent observer of animal life'.[15] His approach for responsible birdnesting required 'moderation and judgement'.[16] Involving the use of a mirror to avoid disturbance to the nest and a spoon or spiral scoop to remove eggs safely, ETW's method also avoided taking set eggs which could be detected through their opacity, and ensured that some eggs were always left in the nest for hatching. By adopting this approach, repeat visits could be made to the nest, allowing observations to be recorded on the time taken to hatch the eggs, the number of broods reared and the rate of growth of the fledglings. To encourage the take-up of responsible birdnesting, ETW shared a list of observations that he compiled with his son Ted. These recorded the earliest and latest nesting times for seventy-four species of birds found within Cheltenham and the surrounding area. He hoped that they would act as a catalyst for others to verify the records or provide supplementary observations.

He promoted the work of the Society for the Protection of Birds[17]as another way to increase healthy interest in the lives of birds, and he supported the levying of a £1 fine (per egg taken) to protect a list of already threatened species in Gloucestershire.[18] As a scientist, he repeatedly emphasised the importance of proper rigour, including 'diligent notetaking, even of the most trivial details'[19] to ensure the systematic recording of every observation, noting the exact time, place and other factors of relevance. 'It is seldom that one individual can follow a process through from beginning to end', he cautioned. 'But faithfully recorded glimpses, if put together, will often complete the picture'.[20]

In an age when voices urging wildlife conservation were rarely heard, ETW's views were probably largely ignored or dismissed. Nevertheless, his insights into the global problem were picked up to some extent.[21] Inevitably, he exercised greatest influence in this field on those closest to him, especially Ted, with whom he shared his love of natural history. Ted himself became celebrated as a wildlife conservationist when, in 1905, he campaigned against the practice of boiling penguins for their oil, particularly on Macquarie Island, at the annual general meeting of the Royal Society for the Protection of Birds (RSPB) and in an address to the International Ornithological Congress. ETW's legacy as a conservationist continued through his son, and, through Ted, inspired the development of Sir Peter Scott into one of the twentieth century's most important conservationists.[22] While it is disappointing to recognise how many of ETW's dire warnings have come true in the modern era, the positive actions, which he urged should be taken to address the crisis, still remain valid.

15
Res Non Verba (1894-9)

Wilson family motto – Severn water – Delancey Hospital Wilson Block –
Diphtheria Block – Cookery School – Sad and anxious times

'... all who have the true interests of Cheltenham at heart will agree with us,
that the drinking water of a town in our position must be above suspicion'.
~ ETW ~

AFTER ETW'S UNCLE, THOMAS Bellerby, died in Philadelphia in 1865,
he described him as a 'great favourite'[1] and, later, proudly displayed in
his study a framed chart of the resolutions[2] passed by the Entomological
Society of Philadelphia[3] in tribute to his uncle. Apart from sharing the
same profession and a similar passion for natural history, both men, it
seems, were kindred spirits, especially in terms of putting into practice
the Wilson family motto 'Res non verba' (meaning 'deeds, not words'),
known to be Thomas Bellerby's favourite motto. The following comments,
made by the Society about his uncle, also seem appropriate for ETW:

> In human character greatness of the very highest type consists in an
> enlightened judgement and a good heart; not in the faculty or the
> disposition for making personal demonstrations. The demonstration of a
> great mind shows itself by good and great deeds performed silently and
> with the least possible ostentation; good and great deeds whose influence
> may last through all time without any alloy of evil.[4]

At the beginning of 1894, one of the 'good and great deeds',
which ETW recognised required urgent action, concerned the possible
introduction of water from the River Severn to meet the town's drinking
water supply. The impact of recent drought conditions, coupled with new
legal obligations, placed increasing pressure on Cheltenham's already
dwindling supply and reservoir levels. Once again, the question arose
about the suitability of the Severn to meet the potential shortfall; but
now, the political situation had changed since the question was last given

serious consideration, back in March 1877. Dr Thomas Wright, the first Medical Officer of Health, had died ten years earlier. Significantly, his replacement, Dr John H. Garrett, a chemist by training, shared the same view as Mr G. H. Ward-Humphreys (ETW's least favourite member of the Town Council) that the Severn contained '... water which may be drunk without the slightest danger to health'.[5] After hearing this, ETW wasted no time in galvanising local opposition. He consulted medical colleagues and produced a memorial, signed by twenty-two doctors and surgeons and four retired military surgeons, which stated:

> It is an undeniable fact that the Severn is a navigable and sewage-polluted river. The evidence taken before the Royal Commission on the Metropolitan Water Supply goes to show that water so polluted can be purified; but that this can only be done by the most efficient filtration: a result exceedingly difficult to attain. For, even in London, where the best supervision is obtainable, this filtration is sometimes carried out in a way which the Commission describes as "quite inadequate".[6]

Although medical opinion was divided on the issue, the Town Council endorsed Dr Garrett's recommendation. ETW was outraged, accusing Dr Garrett of pronouncing 'clarified sewage as "not so bad"'; and commenting that with a weak Town Council in charge it meant that 'the Severn was mixed with our pure Hill springs and "half and half" was henceforward to be our drink forever'.[7] It was not until September 1896 that the Severn water was suddenly turned on for use in the town and, a year later, it was made permanent.[8] ETW maintained pressure on the authorities to account for their actions, for example by writing the following letter on 15 December 1896:

> I should like to nail one coin to the counter which has too often been in circulation, viz., the assumption that those who object to the use of water from a navigable river, into which several towns pour their sewage, expect a catastrophe whenever that water is drunk. They do not expect any such thing, but they know that the use of such water is attended with dangers, which may come suddenly and without warning, and they consider such water nasty, whatever filtering processes it may go through. That the Severn water, which Cheltenham people were driven to drink in a time

of drought, was the "purest distributed to the Borough during the year" requires explanation; and that it caused no disease during the two or three months of its use, does not by any means confirm the arguments of those who (in the face of its condemnation by two Parliamentary Committees in succession) advocated its introduction into Cheltenham. We were told when the Severn water was turned into the mains, but we have not been told that it has been turned off, though the reasons for its supply to the town have ceased to exist. It is due to the very large number of persons who object to this source of supply, that they should in future be informed on these important points.[9]

Yet it was to no avail, and there was no turning back. While there has been some later criticism of ETW for the ethics of leading a group of doctors to publicly counter the advice given to the Town Council by their own Medical Officer of Health,[10] the key issue at that time still concerned scientific proof of the authorities' ability to purify polluted water through reliable filtration methods.

~~~

M ORE POSITIVE PROGRESS WAS achieved on 22 July 1895 when the Wilson Block of the Delancey Hospital, a wing of the main building, was officially opened. Named after Charles Wilson (no relation to ETW), the chairman of the trustees, who donated £1,000 to the cost of the £4,000 building, it comprised two wards for the treatment of typhoid and scarlet fever patients. By now, ETW was the sole survivor of the original trustees. In a speech summarised by the *Cheltenham Chronicle* at the opening ceremony, he proudly outlined the hospital's main achievements to date:

During the twenty-one years of its existence there had been thirty-one outbreaks of small-pox in the town, each one of which might have been the cause of a serious epidemic; but as the patients had been taken to the hospital, the whole number of cases had been forty, while only five of them had proved fatal. It was a significant fact that during the twenty years previous to the establishment of the hospital there had been 114 deaths from small-pox in Cheltenham. With regard to the prevention of the spread of zymotic diseases, he mentioned that since the Notification Act[11] had been in force, out of 905 cases which had occurred in the town during the four years, about 706, or 78 per cent., had been isolated in the Delancey Hospital. Between 1878 and 1894 only thirty-six deaths from those causes had occurred in the town, twenty-nine of them being in the hospital. But during the sixteen years previous to the period mentioned there had been 363 deaths. Speaking of the advantages of the treatment in the hospital, he showed that the mortality there was very small, as during the past eighteen years it had only been 2.1 per cent. of the cases sent in. In all 1,415 patients had been treated in the hospital since its foundation, and they had borne testimony to the kindness and skill with which they had been treated (applause).[13]

A few years later, on 9 March 1898, there was even more to celebrate when the final piece of the Delancey jigsaw was put in place - the opening of a new block of buildings for the treatment of diphtheria. Costing approximately £2,500, the block was opened with a specially-designed key, 'an artistic piece of work in steel and copper'.[13] For ETW, the event marked the culmination of twenty-five years of tireless management of the hospital. The new block, constructed with Stonehouse red brick and Bridgwater roof tiles, made provision for 100 additional beds. Internally, all mouldings and dust-harbouring receptacles had been removed and the walls covered in duresco (a type of resin) in order to prevent the transmission of germs. Once again, these new facilities provided considerable success in the fight against infectious disease (see Appendix 3).

For more than thirty years, ETW had fulfilled the role of honorary secretary to the trustees. As the *Cheltenham Examiner* acknowledged, 'to him really belonged the credit of the erection of the new diphtheria block, he having guided and directed the whole of the work'.[14] In his speech, ETW recalled that diphtheria was not a common ailment when the hospital was first designed. At that time, diphtheria appeared to affect only those living in the country but, in later years, had inexplicably become more prevalent in towns.

The new facilities were unusual in that they had been established entirely by voluntary effort, in contrast to equivalent hospitals supported out of the rates. However, the funding model was not straightforward since the hospital acted only partly as a charity. While it was ETW's aim that the poor should not be charged at all, this was only achievable through a generous subscription list. For this reason, he encouraged the local townspeople to think that in subscribing to the Delancey they were benefiting the whole community, not just themselves. He commented:

> To a subscriber who either came in himself or sent his children in, it ceased to be a charity, because he certainly got his money's worth; and it would pay anyone who lived in the neighbourhood to subscribe to the hospital as a matter of insurance against infectious disease because non-subscribers coming in were required to pay double fees. But a subscriber who neither came in himself nor sent a patient in was doing a real charity, because the trustees did not declare dividends nor did they wish to make money. They wished simply to make both ends meet, and the more money received by way of subscription the lower the terms they were able to charge the poor.[15]

~~~

ANOTHER GOOD CAUSE THAT ETW supported around this time was the local School of Cookery. Although an earlier school was established in the late 1870s, it only achieved short-lived success. A new school, first proposed in 1891, opened at new premises at 9 St James's Square on 27 January 1899 with the aim 'to give girls of all classes some opportunity of systematic education in much of the work they would have to perform throughout their lives: the government, management and actual work of their homes'.[16] Catering mainly for elementary school children and students from private schools, including the Ladies' College, the facilities included a fifty-four-seat lecture hall which was used for teaching a curriculum covering cookery, laundry, household management, dressmaking, millinery, and confectionery. Public cookery demonstrations were also given on a weekly basis, and produce offered for sale at discounted rates. Previously, ETW had officiated at the school's prize-giving event, at which he drew attention to the number of cases that had been referred to him as a result of bad cooking.[17] 'Good cookery was most essential to health', he commented, 'an enormous amount of illness arising in the first place from indigestion'.[18] He particularly promoted the school's class for invalid cookery.

~~~

N OW, IN HIS EARLY sixties, there were signs that ETW's health was beginning to fail. Following a Friends in Council meeting on 1 May 1894, his pulse dropped to forty and he experienced difficulty in breathing, though a morphia injection provided quick relief. Nevertheless, ten days later, he was well enough to travel to Cambridge to see Ted receive the first part of his Natural Science Tripos degree. Then, in January, there was worrying news about Nellie who developed pleuropneumonia whilst working in a London hospital. During one of the coldest winters on record, ETW and Mary rushed to her side. Fortunately, her condition improved, and ETW was able to marvel at the 'huge masses of ice'[19] drifting on the Thames below London Bridge. Later, after Nellie had recovered, she went to work in Leicester Royal Infirmary but, in February 1896, contracted enteric fever (typhoid) and, the following month, died as pneumonia set in. It was the family's wish that she should be buried next to Gwladys in the churchyard of St Peter's, Leckhampton after permission was granted by the Medical Officer of Health to allow the body to be removed. ETW commented, '... it was a sad, sad time'.[20]

A further shock occurred on 17 December when the *Westal* household was wakened around 6 a.m. by a powerful earthquake, causing them to wonder 'how the delicate tracery of the [Cheltenham] College chapel had stood the strain'.[21] Despite these recent unsettling events, the family Christmas was celebrated with the usual jollity, ETW memorably producing a fine Christmas card for Mary, to whom he once wrote in a poem, 'If Mother Xmas walks this earth this surely must be She'.[22]

Further anxiety arose when Ted's health began to deteriorate. He had been working at the Caius Mission, located in the centre of the Battersea slums. Here the educated classes of Victorian England strove to better the lot of the working-class slum dwellers - similar to the modern practice of 'taking a year off' to go and 'do good' in the Third World. While Ted put his poor health down to the effects of London pollution, eventually it became clear that it was of a more serious nature. In June 1897, when ETW went to visit Ted in Battersea, he probably thought it was down to Ted's gruelling schedule, which had recently increased through having to deputise for the Mission Warden whilst he was away. It was not until the

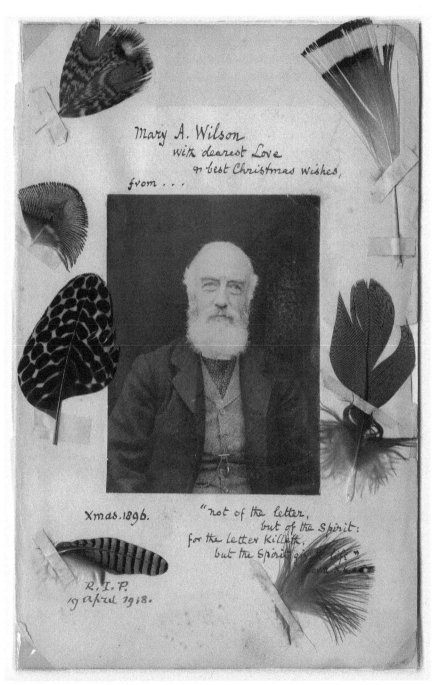

Example of a Christmas card made by ETW for Mary.

beginning of March 1898 that all became clear. ETW was startled when Ted suddenly appeared at *Westal* with a temperature of 38.3°C (101°F). He carried with him a letter from Dr Rolleston, diagnosing that Ted had developed pulmonary tuberculosis and recommending that he should go to Davos in Switzerland for treatment in a sanatorium. In those days, this diagnosis usually meant a death sentence. There was no treatment beyond getting plenty of rest and fresh air. Ted left for Davos on 31 October. 'As the disease had been detected early', ETW commented, 'we had strong hopes of recovery but the possibilities of failure could not but throw a shadow over our Christmas'.[23] While ETW received a letter from Ted complaining about the sheer boredom of the cure,[24] nevertheless, his prayers were answered the following May when his son returned in better health. By the close of the year, however, a different concern arose. 'The Boers also were causing great anxiety at home', ETW wrote, 'and Bernard writes that "Something must be done"'.[25]

16
A Bolt from the Blue (1900-05)

Death of Rathmel – Bernard in the Boer War – Ted on the *Discovery*
Expedition – Sale of *The Crippetts* – British Medical Association
Conference – Sanatorium for Consumptives – Ted's art exhibitions –
Ireland – Death of Charly

'Next came as a bolt from the blue the chance of joining the Expedition which
Captain Scott was fitting out to go to the Antarctic'.
~ ETW ~

THE NEW CENTURY BEGAN with great sadness. ETW's youngest
brother Rathmel died at Cheltenham on 4 January at the age of
fifty-three. After working as a sheep and cattle farmer in Argentina,
sometimes with his brother Harry, where he became horrified by the
levels of drunkenness, he decided to work for the temperance cause when
he returned to England in 1880. For nearly eighteen years, he worked
most successfully[1] as organising secretary of the Salisbury Diocesan
Branch of the Church of England Temperance Society before poor health
forced his resignation. Additionally, there was anxiety of war, following
the intensification of the Second Boer War (1899-1902) since October.
Under-prepared and struggling against the well-armed Boers, it had
started badly for the British forces. The answer seemed to be to fight
back with a larger army. On 7 March, Bernard enlisted as a trooper in the
Yorkshire Yeomanry 66th Company. It was 'a sad and anxious time for
all who had friends engaged in the Boer War', ETW commented, 'and the
early reverses made it doubly so'.[2]

The following month brought some welcome distraction from the
anxiety when the family hired a shop window to watch the first motor
cars race through Cheltenham. The occasion was the Thousand Miles' Run
organised by the Automobile Club of Great Britain and Ireland to promote
motor vehicles and prove their capabilities to withstand the rigours of
long journeys. ETW marvelled at the large Daimlers and 7-horse power
Peugeots which careered through the Montpellier area of the town, careful

not to exceed the regulation 8 m.p.h. town-speed limit. The cars stopped at the Winter Garden where they were exhibited to a 2,000-strong crowd.

Then, in June, ETW commented that 'a bolt came from the blue in the shape of a letter from Ted'.[3] Earlier that month, Ted had been astonished to receive two letters from ETW's old Oxford friend Dr Philip Sclater (1829-1913), now Secretary of the Zoological Society of London, encouraging him to apply for the post of junior surgeon and zoologist for the forthcoming British National Antarctic Expedition that was being organised by Sir Clements Markham, President of the Royal Geographical Society (RGS).[4] Nothing could have been further from Ted's mind. He was only just reaching the point of fully recovering from tuberculosis; the thought of going to Antarctica instead must have seemed extraordinary to him. Shortly after completing his MB degree,[5] he wrote to his father:

> It's an expensive thing this M.B., but I'm glad at last to have it in safe keeping, and if it lands me at the South Pole it will be well worth the expense. I am going for it for all I know because it is obviously a golden opportunity.[6]

At this stage, Ted's knowledge of Polar exploration was probably less extensive than his father's. ETW's understanding of the practicalities of exploring the *Terra Australis Incognita*, or Unknown Southern Land, was fairly advanced in view of his early friendship with Dr David Lyall (1817-95), the Scottish-born Royal Naval surgeon and naturalist who came to retire in Cheltenham in 1878. As Assistant Surgeon on HMS *Terror* during the British Antarctic Expedition (1839-43) under Sir James Clark Ross, Lyall had contributed to one of the greatest early voyages of exploration to the Southern Continent. His ship, together with HMS *Erebus*, were the first to penetrate the Antarctic pack ice and enter what was thought to be a lagoon (later named the Ross Sea) and then witness the Great Ice Barrier (later renamed the Ross Ice Shelf).

Living at 1 Priory Parade (now 24 London Road), very close to ETW's practice when it was at The Priory, Lyall shared much in common with ETW, especially medicine, science and natural history. Their friendship was probably also strengthened through the fact that Lyall knew Charly, having accompanied him during the North American Boundary Commission work in 1858. Of greatest delight to ETW was the

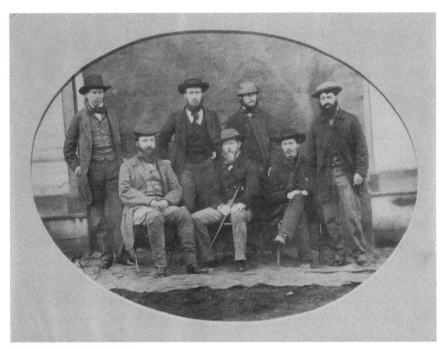

Officers of the Oregon Boundary Commission, c.1858 (David Lyall seated front row on left; Charly seated front row on right)

opportunity to hear detailed accounts of Lyall's remarkable journeys to the Antarctic and Arctic regions, including the story of how the *Terror* and *Erebus*, under sail only,[7] succeeded in breaking through the pack ice into the "lagoon" of open water after repeatedly striking the ice at the same point for a week. Lyall also spoke about the significant achievements of Ross's expedition: the discovery of Victoria Land, McMurdo Sound and the two volcanoes, Mount Erebus and Mount Terror, named after both ships. Perhaps Scott would name a new geographical feature after Ted[8] in the same way as Ross had named the Lyall Islands (167° 20' E) for ETW's friend in 1841.

ETW's knowledge of Lyall's experience increased his fears for Ted's safety. Lyall had encountered many fierce gales and high seas in the Southern Ocean, the worst of which caused the two ships to collide and the *Erebus* - after losing some rigging - to nearly smash into a huge iceberg; but it was Lyall's contributions to science that also impressed ETW. Lyall's illustrious career as a botanist placed him on a par with his close friend, Sir Joseph Hooker. Yet, because Lyall never recorded his memoirs for posterity, his remarkable contributions - except through some recent articles[9] - have largely been overlooked.

~~~

A GENERAL ATMOSPHERE OF sadness returned to pervade the family at the end of September when Mary, much against her own wishes, decided to sell the lease of *The Crippetts*.[10] The bailiff, Griffin, had lost the farm large sums of money through his 'drunken carelessness',[11] and his negligence meant that it had become unsustainable. On being sent to Andoversford to sell some pigs at this time, Griffin got so drunk that he fell out of the trap on his way home and hit his head. It ensured that he was not re-employed by the new owners and he had to break rocks for a living instead. Devastated by the loss of *The Crippetts*, Ted suffered another drawback around this time. Having recently been appointed to the post of Junior House Surgeon at Cheltenham General Hospital, he cut himself in the course of his medical duties and developed blood poisoning and an abscess of the axilla. ETW helped to drain out the pus under ether from his armpit, but Ted was soon forced to resign from his post.

~~~

A S THE YEAR DREW to a close, ETW's attention was drawn to the plans being made for the BMA to hold its Annual Meeting in Cheltenham next summer. 'The Presidency had been offered to me', he commented, 'and I should have liked to accept it but as a family man I did not consider that I was justified in undertaking the expense'.[12] Instead, his friend, Dr G. B. Ferguson (1843-1906), a surgeon at Cheltenham General Hospital, was elected as President, while ETW filled the lesser role of President of the Medical Section. Additionally, however, given his considerable knowledge of Cheltenham, he also took responsibility, together with John Sawyer, for producing a guide to the town to support the BMA visit.

~~~

T HE FOLLOWING YEAR, AS the cold Cotswolds winter set in, memories of hot summer days spent in St Petersburg were rekindled when Fan

(Frances B.) Whishaw, one of Mary's relatives, came to stay at *Westal*. Whilst working as a governess Fan wrote novels under the pseudonym of Sinclair Ayden. ETW found her 'a most interesting personality'.[13] Hired in 1894 to look after the children of the Russian Avinoff family,[14] the experience provided her with much of the inspiration for *Rolling-Flax; or Summer Days in Little Russia* which she published in 1902.[15] Shortly after bidding farewell to Fan came the news of the death, on 22 January, of Queen Victoria. Much saddened, ETW went with Elsie to Gloucester Cathedral to attend the memorial service but found they were 'unable to get inside the doors – so great was the crush at every avenue'.[16]

During May, a delightful time was spent with the family. They welcomed back Bernard after eighteen months' campaigning in the Boer War which, memorably, involved him in an (unsuccessful) attempt to capture the elusive Boer general Christiaan Rudolf de Wet (1854-1922). While Bernard had been heavily involved in fighting, ETW noted that his greatest hardships emanated from the vermin attached to his clothes.[17] ETW also closely followed the fortunes of his nephews, Charles Stuart Wilson (1867-1933) and Francis Adrian Wilson (1875-1954) during their wartime service, the latter winning the D.S.O. at Laing's Nek during the First Boer War and then, during the Second, helping to defend the besieged garrison at Ladysmith.

Then, with the imminent departure to the Antarctic, ETW enjoyed a long walk in Cranham Woods with Ted, now accompanied by his new fiancée Oriana Souper (1874-1945), known as Ory, whom he met in Battersea. A fortnight later, ETW went to London to meet Captain Scott (1868-1912), Lieutenant Royds (1876-1931) and Ted's other shipmates on the *Discovery*, then berthed in the East India Docks.

~~~

A T THE BEGINNING OF July, he attended a meeting at the Montpellier Rotunda in Cheltenham to discuss a scheme to build a Free Open-Air Sanatorium for the treatment of consumptive patients among the poorer classes of the three counties of Gloucestershire, Somerset and Wiltshire. Although the tuberculosis *bacillus* was isolated in 1882, finding a cure still proved elusive. Given Ted's near-fatal experience with the disease, the initiative resonated strongly with ETW.[18] What had worked for Ted in Davos, ETW thought, must surely work for others. Besides, as ETW's friend Dr G. B. Ferguson pointed out, the urgency for action was all too clear: while everyone was currently mourning the loss to date of 15,000 lives in the Boer War, tuberculosis was responsible for 'four times as many as that every year'.[19] ETW strongly supported the requirement for a new sanatorium, recalling the time when medics looked at cases of consumption 'with apathy and despair',[20] but now, with greater confidence, in the light of new treatment methods. He commented:

> They did not know exactly how these things acted upon the disease. It was possible that the parasite might be killed by the fresh air breathed, or it was possible that the fresh air gave the human body sufficient power to resist and kill the parasite. But however it was done, there was no doubt about the fact that the treatment did bring about a cure, and therefore they should do what they could to place that treatment within the reach of all. (Hear, hear.) [...] The proposed Sanatorium could not possibly take all the cases which they might wish to send to it. [...] . It was of no use taking in cases that required isolation for any length of time: what they wanted was to get into this institution cases in the incipient stage, and he hoped means would be found elsewhere for isolating the advanced cases. But even if the Sanatorium were restricted to cases in the earlier stage of consumption it would not accommodate half of the possible number of patients, and therefore he should look upon the institution, not as a place for the isolation of those cases, but really as a school for teaching the treatment of consumption - a place where poor people, after they had been there a month or two, would have learnt how to treat themselves, what amount of fresh air, what kind of food, and what habits were necessary for combatting the disease; and if they had healthy homes there would be no difficulty at all in their continuing the treatment away from the Sanatorium. Medical supervision was very necessary until the rules to be observed were learnt, but afterwards the treatment could be as well carried out at home as it could be in any other place. Whatever happened in the future - even if other remedies for consumption were discovered - the Sanatorium would serve a useful purpose in the sense he had described: it would become a great school for teaching the treatment of consumption in the three counties. (Applause.)[21]

The recommendations made by ETW and his medical colleagues were accepted, leading to construction work for the sanatorium to begin two years later. Located in old quarries at Murhill, Winsley (near Bath), it opened in 1905 and was enlarged in 1911. It proved so successful[22] that it continued treating tuberculosis until 1977.

~~~

LESS THAN A WEEK later, on 16 July, ETW hurried to Hilton in Huntingdonshire (now in Cambridgeshire) to attend Ted and Ory's wedding, at which Bernard was the best man. The following day, he revisited the *Discovery*, still berthed in London, this time with members of the wedding party, to further acquaint himself with members of the expedition. Then, on 24 July, he noted:

> Ted and Ory came for their farewell visit and left next day with many
> fervent wishes and prayers for the safety of our dear boy amid all the
> unknown perils which await him. He left in excellent spirits and the best
> of health.[23]

Little time was then left for making final preparations for the four-day BMA conference which began on 30 July. Now representing a membership of 19,000, nearly a twenty-fold increase on the number when its Annual Meeting was last held in Cheltenham in 1837, the BMA event was one of the largest of its kind held in Cheltenham. Copies of ETW's *A Guide to Cheltenham* were handed out to delegates. Tailored to the audience's needs, it covered topics on health, such as the town's immunity from particular disease, and those of general interest, including social, educational, geographical, historical and leisure aspects. Then, on 1 August, as Chair of the Section on Medicine,[24] ETW gave a short address on the value of research in Medicine and Therapeutics. Surprised at the little progress being achieved through research, he commented:

> Curiously enough, at the last meeting of the Association in Cheltenham
> the results of a collective inquiry into the Influenza epidemic of 1836-37
> were presented, and it would be difficult to say even now, after the lapse

British Medical Association.

CHELTENHAM MEETING, 1901.

. A .

Guide to Cheltenham

EDITED BY

EDWARD T. WILSON, M.B., F.R.C.P.,

AND

JOHN SAWYER.

Cheltenham:

NORMAN, SAWYER AND CO., ST. GEORGE'S HALL.

Title page from ETW's Cheltenham Guide.

of sixty-five years, and with a riper experience, that any real addition has been made to the knowledge shown in that report of the cause, the course, or the treatment of the disease.[25]

The conference, he said, would need to make important decisions about the allocation of its funds. 'Shall we', he asked, 'devote them to political ends or to science, to the mere working machinery of the Association or for the advancement of learning?'[26] The answer, he suggested, was to emulate the example of one of Cheltenham's great public health reformers, Dr Henry Rumsey, and use it to support scientific research.

Apart from the business side of the Meeting, a full programme of entertainments was organised. These included an afternoon garden party hosted by the mayor in Pittville Park, attended by an estimated crowd of 1,500, an illuminated *fête* in Montpellier Gardens, and a range of excursions, receptions and dinners. Participants were also encouraged to visit the Delancey Hospital, hailed as 'one of the first, and ... best of its class'.[27] The conference ended in spectacular fashion with a *soirée* at the Ladies' College, to which over 2,000 people had been invited.[28] Fairy lamps lit up the lawns at dusk, while the crowds mingled, marvelling at the interesting demonstrations and exhibits on display: these included liquid air, colour photography, electrical experiments (by the borough electrician Hamilton Kilgour), microscopic slides of malarial parasites in mosquitoes, working models of turbine engines, wireless telegraphy, X-Rays, calculating machines, and drilling instruments. Those who visited the College's observatory were rewarded with good views of Saturn's rings and Jupiter's planets and an 'equally picturesque view of Cheltenham bathed in moonlight'.[29] A concert by Herr Wurm's Viennese White Band was followed by story-telling, musical sketches and dancing which continued until one o'clock. 'Thus ended a meeting which was pronounced a signal success', commented ETW, '- to us it was most enjoyable from the number of interesting people we met ...'.[30] For ETW, the most remarkable individual he encountered was the distinguished Canadian physician William Osler (1849-1919) who stayed at *Westal* during the Meeting and became a trusted, close friend. As a medical man, ETW considered him omniscient 'with wide and noble aims'.[31]

~~~

JUST A FEW DAYS later, ETW's thoughts were directed at Ted who sailed on the *Discovery* from the Solent on 6 August. Many family members did not think that they would ever see Ted again. It is almost impossible to imagine what it must have been truly like to sail towards the unknown and the sort of courage that it must have taken. Even if we were to launch astronauts today for Mars, they would know more about where they were heading and have better communications with the World than the officers and men who sailed aboard *Discovery*. While Ted was sailing south, the perils of the southern continent became even clearer to ETW when, on 11 November, he attended a lecture at the Winter Garden by Carsten Borchgrevink (1864-1934), the Anglo-Norwegian polar explorer.[32] As leader of the British Antarctic *Southern Cross* Expedition (1898-1900) Borchgrevink established a new 'Farthest South' record at 78° 50' South, but the achievement came at a cost. The zoologist of the expedition, Nicolai Hanson (1870-99), died and became the first person to be buried in Antarctica. If ETW thought this was a bad omen, he did not record it, merely expressing satisfaction with the good photographs shown, especially 'the last one representing [Borchgrevink] in full Antarctic dress – standing alone – and labelled "Furthest South"'.[33]

More compelling first-hand accounts took place the following year which helped ETW to start gathering his own thoughts on Antarctica in preparation for his own series of lectures. On 14 February 1902, after dining with Charly at the RGS, he heard George Murray (1858-1911), the keeper of the Department of Botany at the Natural History Museum, then acting as a temporary scientific director to the *Discovery* expedition, read a paper on the expedition's outward journey as far as Cape Town. Prior to the voyage, Ted had worked at the museum under Murray and had even painted some specimens for him.[34] During the expedition he gave Murray some specimens of birds and eggs, collected from South Trinidad, to bring home. Later, on 14 May, ETW and Charly went to see Ted's sketches of South Trinidadian and other southern birds.[35] However, when ETW visited the Natural History Museum the day after Murray's lecture he wondered how secure any specimens would have been kept in the museum's vaults. On this occasion, he was discussing with the curator of the bird collection, Richard Bowdler Sharpe (1847-1909), the 'raids on [his] father's collection of Humming Birds'.[36] It appeared that the ornithologist and bird artist John Gould (1804-81), who had a special interest in hummingbirds, had repeatedly stolen from the museum's collection to add to his own.[37]

In October, while Captain Scott was making final plans for embarking on an attempt with Ted and Ernest Shackleton to reach the Farthest South, ETW was saluting another Captain Scott. The occasion was the Mayoral Banquet held at the Municipal Art Gallery as part of the ceremony for laying the foundation stone of Cheltenham's new Town Hall. ETW was entrusted with giving the toast to 'Our National Institutions'. Among the institutions he celebrated was the army, which, he thought, 'had earned the title gentlemen through [the Tommies'] behaviour to their enemies'.[38] Then there was the navy, whose bravery and resourcefulness had been recently exemplified by the heroics of Captain Percy Scott (1853-1924)[39] of the *Terrible* in the Cape of Good Hope. Realising that the British Army's guns would be out-ranged by the Boer artillery, Scott mounted the ship's 4.7 inch guns on wheels so that the army could deploy them on land.

ETW also spoke about education[40] and religion, noting that the 'great revival in religious matters had borne fruit in the helpfulness of the rich towards the poor; and the clergy of every denomination had won respect by their singleness of aim and devotion of duty'.[41] Lastly, he turned his attention to health, observing the following:

> The town was fortunate in its hospitals (hear, hear). The Delancey Hospital during its 28 years' existence had isolated 68 cases of small-pox and prevented any spread of that disease while the fact that its scarlet fever mortality had been two during that time showed that it had no need to import the new German serum (laughter and applause).[42]

Then, on 2 November, Captain Scott, Ted and Shackleton set off on the expedition's Southern Journey with nineteen dogs and five sledges, hoping to explore as far as 85° South. Less than two weeks earlier, ETW gave an illustrated paper on 'Antarctica' for the CNSS, with slides borrowed from the RGS. Outlining the plans, questions and conjectures of the current phase of Antarctic Exploration, he began:

> I propose to consider what is at present known of the least explored portion of the globe, of the aims and objects of those who are content

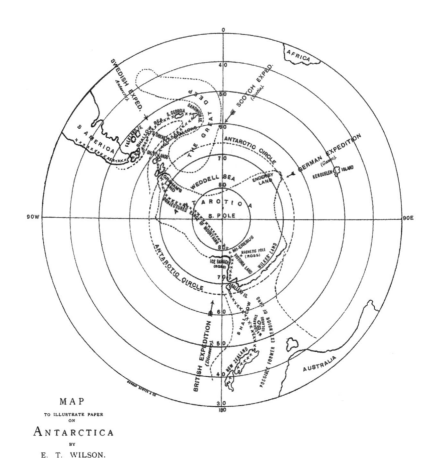

MAP
TO ILLUSTRATE PAPER
ON
ANTARCTICA
BY
E. T. WILSON.

Map of Antarctica showing the proposed routes of the European expeditions including Discovery, from ETW's paper.

"To reside
In thrilling region of thick-ribbed ice;
To be imprisoned in the viewless winds,
And blown with restless violence round about
The pendent world".[43]

Unbeknown to ETW, the above quotation he used from Shakespeare's *Measure for Measure* was particularly apt for the three explorers who were about to experience severe blizzards, difficult surfaces and temperatures of -19°C (-2.5°F). It also reflected the significant challenges faced, earlier, by Ted as the expedition's artist when learning how to paint as the *Discovery* rolled in 40 feet high waves. Drawing on one of Ted's letters, ETW proceeded to give the following example of 'a landsman's recent experience':

> Painting under these circumstances is trying - a bird, for instance, which is swinging through 30° every few seconds; things won't stay as you put them, your water is hung on a hook, your paper pinned to a board, and you hold your paint box; you yourself are wedged into the bunk cupboard and kept there by a boot on the chest of drawers opposite. You put your paint-box down to settle a wing for the thirtieth time when down it rattles and the paints go all over the cabin; you jump to save the paint-box and the corner of your board tilts the water tin off its hook and it empties into a drawer full of clean drawing paper, while a running drip takes the opportunity of coming from the skylight on the painting of the bird you are doing. Everything is at such close quarters and everything trying to balance is with but indifferent success. Our record roll was 56°.[44]

Despite the conditions, while Ted was able to produce technically flawless and aesthetic masterpieces of fine art, equally important, both for ETW and his son, was to achieve important scientific work. ETW commented:

> So long as they can carry forward the lamp of knowledge and discovery into the dark places of the earth and bring back results which will be of service to mankind.[45]

Knowing what scientific achievements the *Discovery* Expedition had made and whether the explorers had set a new 'Farthest South' record were two questions ETW would not know the answer to for nearly eight months. His more immediate question though concerned Ted's safety and well-being. At Christmas, ETW commented that while they drank 'to absent friends' they 'didn't realise the hardships [that] dear Ted was undergoing in his struggle towards the pole'.[46] Nor did ETW know that just over a week before, on 16 December, Ted had been in happy spirits, drinking to his father's birthday and sending him 'good wishes from the south'.[47] Finally, at the end of January, came definite news that all was well. Ory had travelled to New Zealand hoping to meet Ted on his return from the south, only to discover that the *Discovery*, still trapped in ice, had been delayed for another year. While they had not reached the Pole, letters from the relief ship gave satisfactory reports.

Although ETW was disappointed at having to wait another year before the *Discovery* could be released from the ice, he was able at least, on 10 June 1903, to attend Sir Clements Markham's lecture at the RGS, where glowing reports were given on the expedition's first year, the aims of which were:

> ... to study the nature of Ross's great ice barriers; if possible, to discover land to the Eastward; secure various scientific results during the voyage and in Winter quarters; and from Winter quarters to explore the volcanic region, and to make discoveries to the South and inland to the West.[48]

As ETW sat listening to Sir Clements comment about how the expedition had exceeded expectations he was then thrilled to hear him remark that Ted's work on vertebrates was 'exceedingly valuable' and would likely form one of the highlights of the expedition.[49] Sitting next to the father of Louis Bernacchi (1876-1942), the expedition physicist, ETW also shared his companion's pride when it was reported how Mr Bernacchi ascertained the temperature and salinity of seawater at various depths and made other observations using his magnetic instruments and electrometer.[50] However, for ETW, the climax of the lecture came when Sir Clements read the following report of the Southern Journey:

> Captain Scott established a depôt sixty miles to the south in a journey of ten days, from Sept. 23 to Oct. 4, when there was a heavy gale, and the thermometer fell to 51 deg. On Nov. 1 he started with eighteen dogs, accompanied by Lieut. Shackleton and Dr. Wilson. A supporting sledge under Lieut. Barne went as far as the first depôt. At first all went well, but after a fortnight the dogs got weaker and weaker, and a long tract of soft snow had to be crossed, which occupied them for thirty days, bringing the sledges up in relays. Practically the dogs became useless. The explorers had to do all the work themselves. But, nothing daunted, the gallant men pushed onwards, lightening the weight by leaving a depôt in 80 deg 30 min S. They reached 82 deg 17 min S [then the 'farthest south' reached].

On their return Lieut. Shackleton broke a blood-vessel, and was only just able, owing to his extraordinary pluck, to keep up with the sledge; while Scott and Wilson, suffering from snow-blindness and hunger, dragged the sledge back, 240lb each, and reached the ship on Feb. 4, after an absence of ninety-four days. They must have gone over 981 statute miles. The story would be told by Scott himself - a story of heroic perseverance to obtain great results; a story which was unmatched in polar annals. It would tell of new geographical facts and deductions of intense interest; of a new and hitherto unknown world in the far south, reached with such extreme difficulty ....[51]

In fact, the story was first told to the British public by Shackleton who had been invalided home. On 8 January 1904, he gave a lecture at the RGS, which Pollie attended, reporting to her father that Shackleton 'was loud in [his] praises of Ted'.[52] Like Ted, however, ETW was disappointed with aspects of Shackleton's character. Recalling Shackleton's later lectures in 1909, he noted there was 'scarcely a word in his lectures of Scott to whom he owed nearly all he knew and probably his life besides, or of any of his former messmates on the Discovery'.[53]

When, on 3 May 1904, ETW came to give his next lecture, this time on the 'Antarctic Experiences of the Discovery' to his beloved Friends in Council, there was considerably more material upon which he could draw. Thereafter, he continued to glean more knowledge of Antarctic exploration, for example, in August, when he spent a stimulating week at the Meeting of the British Association, held at Cambridge. Here he stayed in a room (just below Ted's when he was a student) at Caius College and heard Dr William Speirs Bruce (1867-1921) give an account of the Scottish Antarctic Expedition. Whilst still at Cambridge he also contributed the latest updates from the Discovery Expedition through letters he had just received from Ted.

Nevertheless, of greatest fascination for ETW during this week was to hear distinguished scientists such as William Thomson, Lord Kelvin (1824-1907), Lord Rayleigh (1842-1919),[54] and Sir Oliver Lodge (1851-1940), discussing the latest theories on the constitution of Matter. Despite the seriousness of the conversations, there was still opportunity for some amusement: this was provided by Francis Longe,[55] ETW's old friend who, he remembered, made 'mud pies in a footbath to illustrate the throwing off of the moon from the earth', adding laconically that 'it was sad for the undergraduate's swell carpet when rotation began'.[56] At the reception at Trinity College he met Arthur Balfour (1848-1930), then Prime Minister, who had given the Meeting's presidential address. Apart from Balfour's 'particularly winning' smile, ETW was 'struck by the firm grasp of his huge hand and the large scale of his features'.[57]

After the euphoria of Cambridge, September provided opportunity for great celebration: the *Discovery* arrived back, docking at Portsmouth, where Ory and Lily went to greet Ted. Two days later, ETW noted:

[Ted] was once more amongst us looking the picture of health and much bronzed. We at once took a photo of him - and it was indeed a treat to hear him tell of all the terrible sufferings and perils which he had undergone.[58]

A few days later, they congregated at East India Dock, where the *Discovery* was now berthed. ETW had long talks with the officers and crew, and attended a celebratory lunch hosted by the Royal Society and the RGS, with several admirals. There, he sat next to the Irish seaman Tom Crean (1877-1938), whom he found 'rather silent and subdued by his surroundings ... [noticing] that he drank his champagne with the greatest discretion'.[59] In the evening, he attended another celebratory dinner. This was hosted by the RGS at the Criterion Restaurant where Clements Markham and several admirals, including Admiral Sir Lewis Anthony Beaumont (1847-1922) and the Arctic explorer of the *Fox* fame, Sir Leopold McClintock (1819-1907), gathered as part of 275 invitees, with Ted as one of the guests of honour. The *Morning Post* noted:

Immediately behind the President's seat stood a glass case containing a splendid specimen of the emperor penguin – one of the zoological treasures secured by the expedition ...In the centre of the chairman's table stood a model, roughly but not unpicturesquely, executed in sugar of the *Discovery*.[60]

After the dinner, the guests listened to *Home, Sweet Home* 'in a silence that was painful in its impressiveness'.[61] Then, on 26 September, the family hosted a reception in Ted's honour at *Westal* for their friends. 'It was a very pleasant gathering', the *Cheltenham Examiner* reported, 'and the congratulations to the traveller upon his return, and to his wife, who was with him, were warmly given and received'.[62] However, the biggest highlight of the event was an exhibition in the library at *Westal* of thirty-five of Ted's water-colour sketches which conveyed 'a more vivid impression of the marvellous scenes depicted than mere words could give'.[63]

Soon afterwards, Ted's stay at Cheltenham was cut short since he needed to work on the expedition collections in the Natural History Museum, amongst them the first exciting scientific specimens of emperor penguin eggs and chicks. He was also soon organising, with Reginald Skelton (1872-1956), who had been the main photographer on the expedition, an exhibition of pictures at the Bruton Gallery in London. ETW attended the exhibition when it opened on 7 November, coinciding with Captain Scott's expedition lecture at the Royal Albert Hall, which ETW and Mary attended in the evening. Ted's exhibition was a huge success, crowds of people having to be turned away from the door. The exhibition's display of the first images of emperor penguin chicks was particularly popular, starting a long fascination amongst the British public. The exhibition arrived in Cheltenham's Town Hall in February 1905, where large crowds once again lined up to see it. While it was one of the most popular exhibitions ever held in Cheltenham, ETW noted how poorly the publicity had been handled:

> Everything had been neglected and put off to the last moment by the manager ... - and on the day of opening 27 February I was sent 100 cards to address to any likely people inviting them to the opening ceremony at 2 p.m. - Even Mr James Winterbotham was only asked in the morning to make an opening speech on the occasion. [...] A few adverts only had been got out and many missed the exhibition from not hearing about it until all was over.[64]

Despite this and the added problem of poor lighting, ETW was pleased that 'the subjects were so novel and the colouring so good that [the pictures] excited a great deal of admiration'.[65] Now, with its connections to Ted, Cheltenham developed an appetite for things Antarctic, with *Westal* a focal point. Captain Scott, who was engaged on a national speaking tour, stayed there in early December 1904, lecturing in Cheltenham twice on 10 December and, the following day, getting caught in a snow storm after traveling to Cirencester, so that he returned late to *Westal*. ETW and Mary nevertheless had several interesting talks with him before he left for Dublin. ETW found him to be 'clever, unassuming and amusing' and 'a born leader of men [to whom] Ted ... [and] every member of the expedition' was devoted.[66]

As Ted started the major task of writing up his share of the scientific reports of the expedition, he sent his scientific papers to his father for comment before submitting them for publication, an act which showed the tremendous esteem in which he held him and which also meant that the local Natural Science Society was kept abreast of developments.

~~~

WHILE THERE WAS MUCH to celebrate in 1905, the year also yielded unwelcome experiences. Among these was ETW's narrow escape whilst travelling on a tram with Bernard and Elsie down Cleeve Hill. After the brakes failed the tram started to career down the hill at high speed. Expecting a catastrophe, they braced themselves but by some good fortune the tram kept the rails and eventually ground to a halt at the bottom. In June, another strange incident occurred when a court case was heard at the Gloucestershire Quarter Sessions. It transpired that a thirty-four-year-old woman had entered George's shop in Montpellier Walk on 28 April and asked for a large meat pie and some cakes, claiming it was for Dr Wilson, her employer and a customer of the shop. Ida went to Gloucester to give evidence, and the woman was found guilty and sentenced to two months' hard labour.

In August, ETW was able to escape for a month-long family holiday with Ted and Ory to the South West of Ireland. With resonances of *Crippetts* days, it was to be the last of the great Wilson family holidays, where long days were spent sketching, birds-nesting, botanising and picnicking. The rugged scenery was a refreshing change, and the entire family rejoiced in having some length of time together in the bracing country air. After returning home, ETW became fascinated during the next two months with the possibility that a Roman race-course might once have existed at Cleeve Hill. Later, in 1909, he published research on this, describing how he vividly imagined 'the chariots madly tearing along' on the site of a platform, which he discovered, whilst also acknowledging that further evidence was needed.[67]

Towards the end of October, ETW went to Tunbridge Wells to visit Charly, who was recovering from an operation after being taken ill in June. Only a few weeks earlier, in May, the two brothers had attended a *soirée* at the Royal Society to hear Ted give a lecture on the Antarctic. Yet sadly, by the time ETW arrived at the station, he was met by Charly's eldest son who informed him that Charly had just died. It was a bitter blow, the sadness also bringing back unhappy memories of the Fall of Khartoum scandal in which Charly had been the unfair target for malicious slander. For ETW, Charly was best summed up as 'an indulgent father, a loving brother and the fastest of friends'.[68] He added:

> Thus ended a life of constant work and strain - a noble record of services done for his country, done quietly and without display – rewarded indeed by his Queen and all the learned Societies in the land but much more by the love and devotion of those who knew him best, who had enjoyed his friendship or profited by his help.[69]

As the year drew to an end, now over five years after ETW received Ted's 'bolt from the blue', ETW proudly recorded that Ted received the Polar Medal from the King at Buckingham Palace, whilst also presenting His Majesty with two of his sketches, including one of the recently discovered King Edward VII Land.[70] Nevertheless, while Ted had achieved nation-wide fame, the local press thought Ted's ability to command such an exceptionally large audience in Cheltenham was due in no small part to Ted being the 'son of Dr. E. T. Wilson'.[71]

17
A Museum for the Town (1906–9)

Resignation from Cheltenham Hospital – Campaigning for a Town
Museum – Death of close friends – Failure to revive spa – School of Art
– Revival of Photographic Society – Temperance Movement – Renewed
focus on the Antarctic

*'Our museum should be no curiosity shop, in which dusty specimens of moth-
eaten, ill-stuffed birds and animals, mummy cases, and ancient pickles shock
more senses than one'.*
~ ETW ~

A T SOYER'S PRIVATE HOTEL, located at *Wolseley House*,[1] Oriel Road,
on 26 June 1906, a small group of doctors enjoyed a celebratory
dinner of fine French cuisine. Among the hosts was Dr G. B. Ferguson,
remembered fondly as 'a wonderful raconteur' who enjoyed the daily
habit of coming into the Hospital Dispensary to get a pick-me-up which,
on one occasion, led to an unfortunate incident.[2] As the guests savoured
the delights of various *Hors d'Oeuvres, Crème St Germain, Turbot Cardinal,
Mousseline de Poularde Alexandra, Coquilles de Foie Gras Strasbourgeoise,
Salade Russe*, and *Noisettes d'Agneau Princesse*, followed by *Jambon – Sauce
Cumberland, Mignons de Bordeaux Paysanne, Pêches Melba, Petits Gondolier
d'Anchoix*, they had particular fun when the *Neige Wilson*[3] arrived.[4] As the
occasion marked ETW's retirement from Cheltenham General Hospital,
a connection which had lasted nearly forty-five years, the conversation
and wine flowed freely, lingering over many happy memories and across
decades of the doctors' friendship and teamwork. ETW was in no doubt
that the timing of his resignation at the age of seventy-three was right.
While his colleagues had persuaded him to stay on for two or three years,
his reason for retirement stemmed simply from a desire to 'make way for
younger men',[5] rather than a lack of energy or capability. However, his
close links with the hospital continued, as he not only remained one of the
governors but was also appointed a consulting physician.

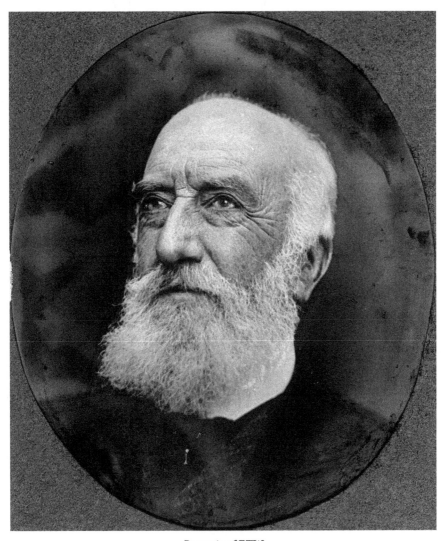

Portrait of ETW.

Following his resignation ETW was able to devote more time to the need for a town museum, a subject which he had already promoted vociferously for fifteen years. Fundamentally, his interest stemmed from a museum's potential contribution to scientific education. While Cheltenham hosts a prestigious science festival today, attracting some of the leading scientists of the day, during the nineteenth century the town seemed to lack a real taste for science, 'the library-proprietors [asserting that] no work of science is ever called for'.[6] ETW encountered this issue too. As President of the Cheltenham Natural Science Society he had attempted to change the culture by instigating a series of first-class lectures on interesting and popular scientific subjects. In 1890 he pleaded:

> There seems even now to be among many people a lingering suspicion of science subjects – a feeling as though it were a little dangerous and perhaps a little wrong to go to scientific lectures. But a prejudice of this kind was bound to die out, and the more the principles of scientific enquiry and the importance of scientific truth were understood by people generally, the greater would be the appreciation of the opportunities which presented themselves for acquiring scientific information.[7]

Nevertheless, despite his best efforts, his attempts ended with limited success. Talks given by distinguished intellects, including the Revd Dr William Dallinger, the geologist Professor William Boyd Dawkins (1837-1929), who gave a talk entitled 'Our early ancestors',[8] and the photographer Eadweard Muybridge (1830-1904), whose talk on 'The science of animal locomotion' was accompanied with 'a succession of magnificent illustrations',[9] attracted disappointingly small audiences. Consequently, ETW suggested adopting a different approach which might help to focus CNSS members' aims. He commented:

> Competition adds keenness and zest to the collector's work, and I cannot help feeling that if some centre, such as a town museum, were in existence, many of us might do more than we have done as yet with a view to stocking it with valuable material.[10]

ETW's vision envisaged organisations such as the CNSS contributing material to the town museum, a place he saw primarily comprising 'local collections, local observations, local lore, and local facts'.[11] In a paper presented in 1891 he elaborated his thoughts further. Steering away from the idea of a museum as an old curiosity shop full of dusty specimens,[12] he stressed the importance of employing a young, energetic curator (not caretaker) - someone, either male or female, who had achieved a course of scientific study with distinction and could shape the museum's development from the beginning, ensuring that a coherent collections policy was rigidly followed. He commented:

'It is [the curator] who must make the dry bones live, as it were, and tell their story; it is [the curator] who must infuse [his/her] own energy into others if [his/her] collection is to grow, and grow it must or it will inevitably die'.[13]

While recognising the necessary constraints, above all his vision emphasised the educational and research value of the institution. He noted:

We shall not go far wrong, then, in insisting that a museum should in a town like Cheltenham, of limited size and limited resources, be *primarily and essentially* a collection of the *local* fauna and flora – with specimens illustrating the geological and archaeological features of the neighbourhood. With a view to rendering the educational value of the local collections more complete a limited – strictly limited and well-chosen – series of type specimens may be added from beyond the local boundaries, but no foreign beast or bird or butterfly which has not a definite educational value should be tolerated. Instruction and research should be the keynote of the collection, the test by which everything should be tried that comes to the curator's hand.[14]

Although ETW's ideas gained some initial support, they also prompted further debate. There was concern, for instance, that the town museum could simply become 'a Natural History mixen'[15] (i.e. dunghill). ETW also feared that it would prove to be too unpopular with ratepayers,[16] although, at that time, the Town Council had the power to provide a museum without consulting ratepayers if expenditure did not exceed a halfpenny rate (then £500). While ETW insisted that a central location was absolutely essential, there were others who felt that alternative (but less convenient) locations such as the Pittville Pump Room, which was then underutilised, should be considered. If natural history was to be its main focus, it was even suggested that a living garden, ideally located in Pittville Gardens, could provide 'infinitely greater educational value than a score of herbariums, howsoever complete or well arranged'.[17] Developing this idea further, it was also suggested that geology could be represented in the gardens in the following way:

... a diminutive duplicate of Leckhampton Hill, made up of actual rock, would much more powerfully appeal to the student than a coloured diagram hung upon the Museum walls.[18]

Yet, ETW remained resolute in his views:

No! the museum should be close to its curator, close to books, close to its students, and not a Sabbath day's journey from all of these and the public if it is to be of any use whatever ....[19]

Although the Town Council adopted the Museums Act in 1899 no significant action was taken to provide a museum. It was not until 1906, seven years later, that ETW could happily announce that he had pledged 'the good offices of the [CNSS] in furthering the development of a Museum'.[20] This paved the way for positive practical steps to be taken. Then, just over eight months later, on 20 June 1907, in the absence of ETW's friend Alderman James Winterbotham, the chair of the Art Gallery and Museum Committee, ETW was given the honour of opening the town's public museum to an invited audience of local leaders from the scientific, literary, artistic and municipal communities. The *Cheltenham Examiner* commented:

... no more appropriate voice could have been secured [in the absence of Alderman Winterbotham] than that of Dr. E. T. Wilson, who, during his long career in the town, has always striven to stimulate its mental energies, and whose interest in Art, supplementing his wide knowledge of scientific subjects, gives him a title to speak about an institution embracing both those interests.[21]

Greatly enthused by the fact that the town was now keeping abreast of 'modern municipal ideas', The *Examiner*, probably had ETW in mind when it suggested that 'the driving force by which public picture galleries and museums are provided must often be sought for rather in individual action and stimulus than in civic zeal'.[22] Comprising a suite of four rooms on the upper floor of the Cheltenham Public Library building, the new museum took over the space previously occupied by the School of Art.

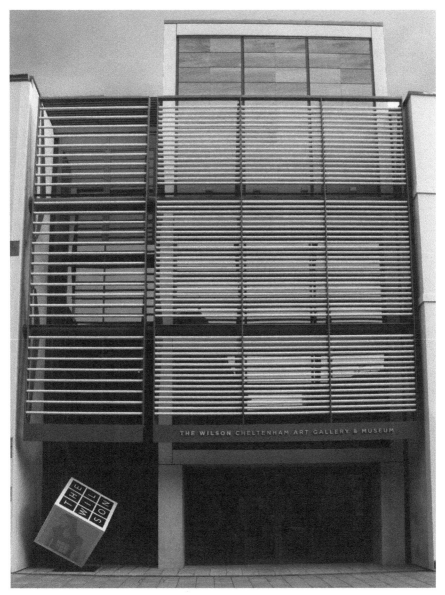

The Wilson Art Gallery and Museum, following its 2013 refurbishment.

Appropriately, the museum and art gallery was renamed The Wilson when, following refurbishment and local consultation for a new name, it was re-opened in 2013.

The opening ceremony took place in the Art Gallery on the ground floor which was connected to the museum by a staircase. In his speech, ETW stressed how indispensable a museum was to any modern town, particularly Cheltenham, given its importance as an educational centre. He then drew attention to how closely-related science and art are. He commented:

> Art, especially on her decorative side, derived some of her deftest touches from the inspiration of Science - from the natural objects about which Science had to teach.[23]

He recalled the original museum exhibits collected by the Literary and Philosophical Institution on the Promenade which, from 1861, were dispersed and formed the nucleus of the museum collection at Cheltenham College. It was there that ETW had provided some voluntary support, which helped to open it up to the general public, although ultimately - given this was only possible for two days a week - a long-term solution needed to be found. ETW also took the opportunity to reiterate some of his thoughts about the role of the museum previously shared in his 1891 paper. He observed:

> Primarily, ... the aim of a museum should be to illustrate the geology, natural history, and antiquities - the characteristic features in fact - of the district in which it [is] placed.[24]

ETW was formally thanked as 'the originator of the Museum' by the Baron de Ferrieres,[25] who commented that '... while many of those in authority had not been very keen for [the museum], his [ETW's] persistency had kept them up to the mark'. [26] Afterwards, ETW conducted a tour of the museum, beginning in a room displaying fossils, shells, geological specimens - some collected by local renowned geologists such as Sydney Savory Buckman (1860-1929) - and Palaeolithic and Neolithic stone and flint tools. Another talking point in this room was the display of a large stuffed female pike, originally found floating on the surface of Dowdeswell Reservoir in 1896, today still one of the museum's most unusual exhibits. ETW then led the party into other rooms displaying examples of sculpture, including plaster reproductions of work by Michelangelo and Donatello; prints and engravings of Cheltenham and Gloucestershire; and decorative art exhibits on loan from the National Art Training School at South Kensington.

In many ways, the day represented the culmination of ETW's lifelong interest and support for museum collections. While always making greatest contribution to museums on his doorstep, he also, where appropriate, made suitable donations to nationally-important collections. Around six weeks before opening the Cheltenham Museum, for example, he travelled to Oxford to present a collection of objects from the Naga Hills region of northeast India to the Pitt Rivers Museum. Comprising various ornaments, including a tapered belt used as defensive armour by high-status Naga warriors, they were originally collected by Robert Gosset Woodthorpe (1844-98), a British army officer in the Royal Engineers, during the 1870s. It seems possible that ETW first met Woodthorpe through Charly given that both officers were RGS members and Royal Engineers. Charly started his career at Chatham in 1863-4 and Woodthorpe did, a year later; and both were involved in survey work and army intelligence. Nevertheless, it is the gift of a chalice,[27] originally owned by Sir Charles Napier (1782-1853), which provides the most tangible link between ETW and Woodthorpe. Although there is no documented evidence for this, it seems likely that when Woodthorpe died in 1898 the Naga collection was passed onto Charly, and then to ETW in 1905 when Charly died. Another possibility is that ETW knew Woodthorpe's brother, J. Dalton Woodthorpe,[28] who lived in Cheltenham and donated some of his brother's collection to the Pitt Rivers Museum in 1916[29] and 1924. What is clear is how much ETW valued the collection; he even had some of Woodthorpe's paintings framed to be hung, presumably at *Westal*.[30] After donating the unique Naga collection, ETW and the curator of Pitt Rivers were pleased that the items now found 'an honourable place'[31] in the museum's cases.

~~~

IN NOVEMBER 1906, MEMORIES of ETW's joyful celebration meal for his resignation were tinged with sadness at the news of the sudden death of Dr Ferguson: the unfortunate surgeon had collapsed with 'scalpel in hand'[32] while performing a critical operation, and the patient had to be saved by an alert house surgeon who quickly deputised for him. More sadness followed with the death of Dorothea Beale (1831-1906), the long-serving Principal of Cheltenham Ladies' College and a great educational pioneer.[33] To ETW she was a close friend, 'always genial and cheerful'.[34] She was one of his patients; and he remembered, once, after he put a thermometer into her mouth that 'she took it out and said "Now tell me all the news" and then replaced it'.[35] Always interested in his daughters, who were former pupils of the College, Miss Beale also showed her support for ETW's efforts to provide the benefits of vaccination in Cheltenham. During the severe smallpox epidemic in Gloucester of 1896, she insisted that all the College workmen were vaccinated at the hospital.[36] At her funeral in Gloucester Cathedral on 16 November, ETW watched a 'sea of sorrowful faces set in the deepest mourning'[37] and wondered who would ever be able to follow in Miss Beale's footsteps. Early in 1907, it was Lilian Faithfull (1865-1952) who was appointed as her successor. Interested in social care provision, she worked with ETW to improve the facilities at the College's private sanatorium[38] on Leckhampton Hill in May 1909.

'Death is indeed busy amongst our friends',[39] ETW reflected. Another good friend, the architect Henry Prothero (1848-1906), a fellow member of Friends in Council, was the next to pass away. ETW thought that he had strained his heart too much through strenuous walks on the continent on account of his 'devotion to art and especially church architecture'.[40] It was fitting that Prothero's funeral was held in the Cheltenham College chapel, one of the great masterpieces of his design work.[41] Then, another hammer blow came with the passing of his oldest friend in Cheltenham, Major Robert Cary Barnard. ETW had much to be thankful for to the veteran of the Crimean War: as founder of both Friends in Council and the Royal Crescent Library, Barnard had contributed greatly to the intellectual life of the town. ETW remembered him tenaciously holding onto his opinions. Although these were often at variance with his friends, it made no difference, and his loss was felt most deeply.[42]

~~~

ALTHOUGH ETW's PERSEVERANCE PAID off with a successful launch of the town museum, this was not to be the case with his efforts to relaunch Cheltenham as a spa. On 20 June 1906, ETW, as one of the members of the Medical Committee, along with the Mayor and the Chamber of Commerce, hosted the inauguration of the Central Spa at the Town Hall. Hundreds of local residents and invited guests from around the country, including members of the medical profession interested in natural mineral water treatment, heard ETW introduce the keynote speaker, Dr James Goodhart (1845-1916), a recognised authority on bath and water treatment. Spirits were high. This was the culmination of years of planning and preparation. Observing that the occasion reminded him of *At Last*, the title of Charles Kingsley's novel set in the West Indies, ETW commented, 'The Central Spa might be regarded as an earnest of what they were going to do'.[43] Reiterating his belief that the experience of Harrogate, Buxton, and Bath showed that there was 'a future for English spas', he added:

> The wells had been thoroughly cleansed and renovated, and their contents carefully analysed by the great authority, Dr Thorp, who was happy to be able to assure everyone that their constituents were identically the same as in the days when they attracted many to the town.[44]

Everything was poised for success. A thousand people had already taken the waters from the Central Spa during the opening six-week period, and there was further potential demand from the expanding population to the north of the town. If anyone else needed convincing, Dr Armstrong of Buxton, a recognised authority on the mineral springs of Europe, opined that 'the Medical profession, particularly in London, would increasingly advise patients to take the cure at Cheltenham and other watering places at home instead of in foreign countries'.[45] Yet ETW's original vision was never realised properly. The Town Council's approach appeared modest and half-hearted.[46] ETW himself put the failure down to poor marketing, while the lack of local enthusiasm provided the final nail in the coffin. The *Cheltenham Examiner* commented:

> For years leading local physicians, notably Dr. WILSON, have been hammering away at the desirability of a Central Spa; and though its movement in that direction has not been marked by the celerity of confident enthusiasm, the Town Council may fairly claim to have kept the object steadily in view. The governing body has been discouraged and thwarted at every turn by a section of the townspeople, and the fact that its own faith perhaps was not robust, did not make for the successful attack of obstacles in the way.[47]

Another attempt to revive the spa was made in March 1907. ETW did his best to address any perceived problems, especially concerning Cheltenham's climate. For a while Cheltenham was promoted as the 'Carlsbad of England' but, ultimately, ETW's ideas remained a pipe-dream.

Some of this disappointment was partly assuaged through the considerable celebration and relief when ETW and Mary became proud grandparents around this time. Earlier, in 1898 and 1905, respectively, Lilian and Pollie had both given birth to sons who died soon afterwards. Now, both were successful in delivering strong and healthy children, Pollie first giving birth to Ruth, and Lilian, a few months later, to Tony. An adoring father, husband and, now, grandfather, ETW revelled in every family gathering and event, assiduously recording with pleasure every birth, christening, and marriage of his ever-expanding family.

~~~

THE REST OF THE year was spent providing support for the School of Art whose premises had now moved from Clarence Street to St Margaret's Road, and conducting some research on the human hand, with special reference to fingerprints.[48] The latter included the challenge of collecting fingerprints of chimpanzee and orangutan, which ETW described as 'mischievous children' after they played pranks in the kitchen at London Zoo while he tried to take their prints.[49] Later, in 1911, ETW tried unsuccessfully to collect fingerprints from Consul, 'the clever chimpanzee' who, he recorded, 'gave a performance, which showed wonderful intelligence and training',[50]. He added:

> He used knife and fork adroitly, unlaced his boots, smoked a cigar which he evidently enjoyed, rode a bicycle in and out of obstacles, but was withal ill-tempered and I could not get a finger print.[51]

After spending time with Scotland Yard police officers involved in the application of the new fingerprints identification system ETW recognised the significance of his research which, later, formed part of their exhibition at White City.[52] Prophetically, he commented:

The importance of identification in the ordinary affairs of life seems not to be realised, otherwise finger prints would be as universal as vaccination, perhaps more so.[53]

His research on the human hand also drew on an unusual condition of syndactyl, the partial webbing of the fingers, which he came across at Cheltenham General Hospital.[54] Despite the handicap, the patient was still able to play the piano.

During 1908, ETW turned listener rather than speaker when he attended a number of interesting locally-held lectures: from General Baden Powell (1857-1941), speaking about the Scout Movement,[55] to Flinders Petrie (1853-1942), the renowned archaeologist, on pre-historic Egypt,[56] and Sir Charles Eliot (1862-1931) who gave a lecture at the Ladies' College on the East Africa Protectorate.[57] Then, at the beginning of 1909, ETW was given the opportunity to reflect on fifty-five years of photography when a heavily-promoted meeting at the Town Hall was held to attempt to revive the Cheltenham Photographic Society, which had recently lain dormant. As the co-founder of the society in 1865, along with Dr Abercrombie, ETW ('for many years the life and soul of the old society')[58] reflected on the changing public attitudes towards photography and its exciting new developments. He commented:

At one time everybody spoke against it as likely to result in the death of art. It was indeed to be regretted that photography had driven the beautiful art of miniature painting from the field; but otherwise it had been a great incentive to art progress and the cultivation of the artistic taste. Think of what it had done for book illustration, and also in providing cheaper productions of the Old Masters for the people in a way nothing else could do. Then there was the fascinating domain of colour photography, in which increasingly beautiful results were being obtained. As a method of illustrating lectures on travel, photographic lantern slides were simply invaluable; and the great use to which photography might be put in education generally was hardly as yet appreciated in this country, though well understood in Germany. In astronomy the sensitive plates had revealed bodies which the eye had previously overlooked. Photography had also revealed the wonders of the microscope. People, who had had to crowd round a microscope to take their turn in seeing a good specimen, could now see it at ease together by means of the lantern. The snap-shotter, too, was ubiquitous; and, finally, photography had been of the greatest possible use to the police. With regard to the future, he believed that the greatest improvements would be made in moving pictures, which when coloured and accompanied by sound reproduction would become the most popular and useful achievement of photography.[59]

Towards the end of the year, in November 1909, ETW turned his attention to a public health issue of increasing concern, that of alcohol abuse. He was asked to give an address at the Town Hall by the Church of England Temperance Society[60] as part of its Great Forward Movement, aimed at increasing the Society's membership throughout the country. While agreeing to advocate sensible temperance, he refrained from promoting total abstinence. The large crowd that gathered to hear ETW's views probably reflected the growing drink-related problems that were now occurring in the town. Recognising that Cheltenham, then with a population of around 50,000, had a licensed premise for every 209 people, ETW suggested displaying a map of the town's drinking places in a prominent location so that the inhabitants could see any progress being made to reduce the large number. Apart from correcting some myths about alcohol and focusing on the importance of educating young people about drink, he also talked about the issue from the medical point of view. He warned:

... nobody saw more of the wretchedness [of] the result of drink than the doctor did: he saw it in every stage, and watched the downward course of many whom he could not save because they would not take his advice. What struck the doctor more than anything else was the excessive ignorance of people, not alone of the poor class, as to what was moderation in drink. He was often astonished, when people came to be examined for insurance, at the answers they gave to the test questions regarding their drinking habits. There were very few who would say they were not strictly moderate - in fact, they all declared and believed they were strictly moderate, whereas an enormous number of them were not so, but were immoderate drinkers, only they did not know it. Though never getting drunk in their lives, yet many of these people were ruining their constitutions just as much as if they got drunk every week. It was this little excess of alcohol taken every day without knowing it was more than they ought to take that was undermining their constitution, and these were the people who, between the ages of 40, 50, and 60, dropped by the way, leaving their children a terrible heritage - because there was no doubt that the drink habit, when it was once attained, was as hereditary as any disease that could be named.[61]

While successfully conveying his thoughts on the subject, however, ETW did not enjoy the meeting itself. Later, he commented:

I was obliged to listen to a tirade of nearly an hour ... on the dangers of even a drop of that deadly poison alcohol. There was no room anywhere for temperance, and my patience was well nigh exhausted.[62]

Although ETW did not dwell on the meeting for long, there was something else at the back of his mind. It was the thought that Ted was to return to the Antarctic. After Ted's meeting with Captain Scott in London on 12 July, when they discussed Ted becoming the Head of the Scientific Staff, ETW commented, 'the die was cast'.[63] Less than a month earlier, Shackleton had returned home triumphantly from his *Nimrod* Expedition (1907-09), having got within 98 miles of the Pole. Hailed as a hero, he then went on a public lecture tour. In early December, ETW heard him speak to a packed house in Cheltenham, the atmosphere 'charged with polar frigidness'.[64] While ETW was not impressed by Shackleton's delivery he was impressed by the quality of the photographs, which included a group of penguins listening to a gramophone.[65] Perhaps he wondered what new discoveries Ted would make about these endearing birds.

18
Contrasts in Antarctica (1910-14)

Portrait by Alfred Soord – *Terra Nova* Expedition – CNSS lectures –
Ponting's pictures – 'The staggering blow' – Memorial for Ted – Visits by
Antarctic veterans – Unveiling of Ted's statue

The tempest raged – in elemental strife
The blizzard shrieked and howled – and Lo!
A solitary tent - (no sign of life)
Lay buried deep in drifts of blinding snow.
~ ETW ~

THE YEAR BEGAN PORTENTOUSLY: during the evening of 22 January, ETW and Mary sallied out to see the Daylight Comet.[1] From a house in Battledown they witnessed its 'silvery tail spread far upwards into the clear frosty sky from the brilliant starlike head'.[2] ETW thought that he had not seen anything as beautiful since observing Donati's Comet, while crossing the English Channel in 1858. During the spring, a growing sense of anxiety emerged about Ted's impending departure for the South. This was felt most acutely by Mary who developed a troublesome nettle-rash as a consequence. It proved so painful that ETW was forced to administer some small doses of morphia to ease her pain.[3]

In April, they visited Pollie and her husband Godfrey at Bushey where, in response to suggestions from the family, ETW sat for his portrait in the studio of Alfred Soord (1868-1915), a favourite pupil of Sir Hubert von Herkomer (1849-1914) who had established a School of Painting there. Famous for 'The Good Shepherd' (also known as 'The Lost Sheep'), which depicts a sheep being rescued on a steep cliff by a shepherd, Soord also painted a portrait of Ted,[4] Mary[5] and his friend, James Batten Winterbotham (1837-1914),[6] whom ETW knew through Friends in Council and their shared interest in art.

ETW's last walk with Ted occurred at the end of May, just prior to Ted's departure to the Shetland islands where he learned about whaling as part of final preparations for the Antarctic expedition. They met again

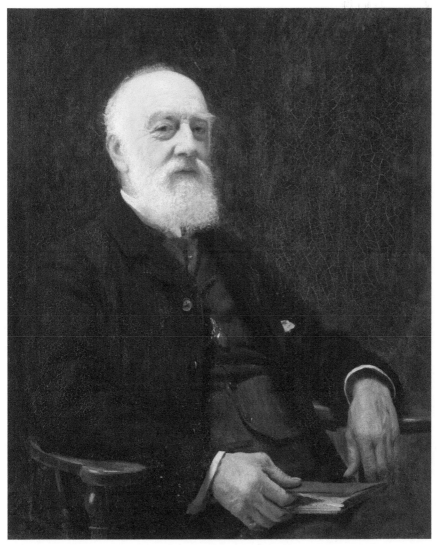

Portrait of ETW by Alfred Soord.

on 15 June in Cardiff, from where the *Terra Nova* sailed. Bands played, crowds cheered, and the ship was accompanied on her way by numerous pleasure steamers, one containing around 750 passengers.[7] Aboard the ship, ETW and Mary watched as proud and anxious parents. Irish Petty Officer Tom Crean (1877-1938), with whom ETW had once dined following the *Discovery* expedition, gave them a tour of the ship.[8] Some unexpected excitement occurred when one of the crew members suddenly

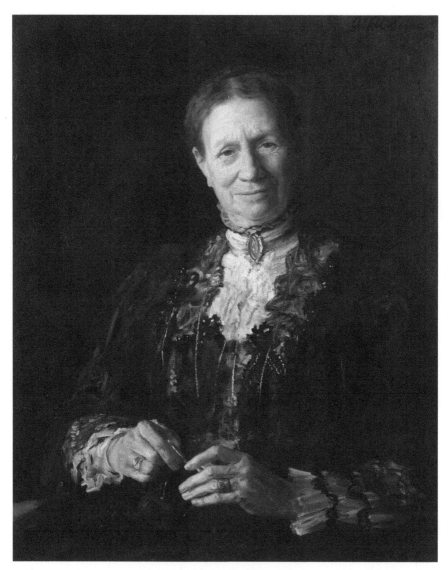

Portrait of Mary by Alfred Soord.

fell overboard as he attempted to fling a coil of rope. ETW was relieved to watch how quickly he swam back to safety.[9] With Ory, they sailed on the ship for some way. ETW commented:

> ...we went out for some 30 miles on the *Terra Nova* and thus had the opportunity of seeing something of the men who were to be Ted's

companions in the South - It was a splendid send off, and many friends were there, among them Hodgson (Muggins) of *Discovery* days who would gladly have been of the company. Ted was very bright but fearfully busy - being wanted in every direction as Head of the Scientific Staff. It was sad to say "good bye" when the inevitable tug appeared which was to take us on shore. We watched the good ship disappear down the coast of Devon and then turned sadly home.[10]

ETW gave Ted a posy of lemon verbena from the garden at *Westal*, which Ted dried to remind him of home. It was the last sight of Ted that his parents would ever have. From that time on, they had to rely on massively-delayed postal communications. Not even the new telephone ETW had installed at *Westal* through pressure from the Ladies' College and Dean Close School, to which ETW provided medical advice, would help the situation.[11] Two days later, ETW wrote to Bernard, expressing hope that both he and Mary would still be alive in two years' time to welcome

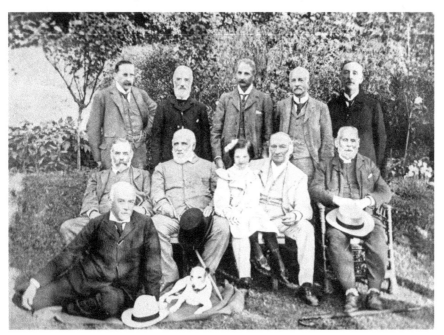

Friends in Council Group Portrait, from 1912 Jubilee book. 12(L-R: Back Row: W. Crooke; ETW; Dr W. R. Buckell; C. Agnew Turner; W. G. Gurney; Middle Row: A. J. de H. Bushnell; Major R. Cary Barnard; J. B. Winterbotham; Rev. W. W. Gedge; Front Row (seated): H. A. Prothero).

Ted home in triumphant success. More immediately, he worried that Ted looked thin and overworked. His hope was that the sea air would soon restore his health.[12] As the *Terra Nova* sailed further south to South Africa, via Madeira, before heading to New Zealand and then onwards into the great Southern Ocean, letters home from Ted, together with copies of his diary entries became less frequent. By the time Ted was enjoying the plum pudding his father had sent with him from Westal to celebrate New Year's Day (22 June) on the Great Ice Barrier, regular communication had ceased.

A few months later, ETW put the final touches to a CNSS paper on the subject of 'Our Inheritance'.[13] He sought to raise interest in the subject and try to answer some of life's big questions: what do we inherit, how do we inherit, and what does it mean for our future lives? It was a topic that had fascinated him even before he collected data twenty-six years previously on the characteristics of the Wilson and Whishaw families which had won him a prize from Francis Galton as part of early research into genetic inheritance. Now, he approached the unpopular subject of eugenics which, he predicted, 'will assuredly have [its] day'.[14] Concerned about lessons from history,[15] the present 'shortage of men fit to fill the responsible civil and military posts' and the fact 'that in Cheltenham, as over the whole country, the poorest of the people are increasing out of all proportion to the better class', ETW did not advocate doing nothing 'for those at the bottom of the social ladder'. He advocated:

> ... steps can and should be taken to find out what [their] inheritance is, and to secure that the environment shall favour and not thwart its development. Every facility should be afforded in our educational system for ability, in whatever form it appears, to take its proper place in the social system ....[16]

Unsurprisingly, around this time, ETW also spoke about the Antarctic. While Ted had recently experienced icy blasts at Cape Evans and was bemoaning the fact that they had not changed their clothes nor had the opportunity to wash since January,[17] ETW was giving a 'splendidly illustrated lecture'[18] in the comfort of clean clothes and the warmth of Dean Close School. Addressing the School Field Club, he focused mainly on the scientific developments recently made by the *Discovery* expedition.

For both he and Ted, scientific success was of paramount importance. On the day[19] Scott sent a telegram to Ted formally confirming his position as Chief of the Scientific Staff for the *Terra Nova* expedition, Ted had written to his father:

> No one can say that it will only have been a Pole-hunt, though that of course is a *sine qua non*. We must get to the Pole; but we shall get more too … We want the Scientific work to make the bagging of the Pole merely an item in the results.[20]

In February 1911, Scott had already received the bitter blow that Roald Amundsen (1872-1928) had just been spotted in the Bay of Whales, an inlet in the Great Ice Barrier. If the Scott expedition was to be the first to reach the Pole, then from this point on their chances of success were greatly diminished. In Ted's opinion, if Amundsen and his men could survive the winter they would be able to travel faster to the Pole with over 100 dogs to support them. For Ted and ETW, however, it was the scientific work, which Ted had travelled nearly 10,000 miles to complete, that was of greatest importance.

The Dean Close students listened intently to ETW's description of the hazardous conditions in which the men lived, including the need to take regular (two-hourly) magnetic readings over a two-year period in a small hut, sometimes only reached after fighting their way through severe blizzards. There was also 'the curious mental state which they developed, and of the method they devised for drawing rations, not being able to trust themselves when food was scarce'.[21] Equally memorable was ETW's descriptions of penguins: while he compared the 2 feet-high king penguins to dolphins when swimming in the sea, he said they look more like nuns on the land as they 'walk twenty or thirty abreast in one direction, stare, and walk back again'.[22] Nevertheless, it was his detailed account of emperor penguins which held centre-stage. When ETW gave his 1902 lecture on the Antarctic he highlighted the absence of knowledge about their nesting place.[23] Around eight years later, how proud he felt, thanks to his son's pioneering scientific notes of the breeding cycle of the emperor penguin, that he was now able to describe the remarkable process in which the birds come onto the ice for the sole purpose of laying their eggs: how these are kept warm after being pushed onto the penguins' feet and insulated by a feather flap; and how the penguins stand on the ice, having to endure the extremes of the Antarctic winter until the eggs are hatched.

In that lecture, ETW had also anticipated the purpose for which his son was to undertake an even more hazardous expedition, later described by Ted as 'the weirdest bird-nesting expedition that has been or ever will be'.[24] This was to visit the breeding ground of emperor penguins in order to collect their eggs. ETW had written:

> ...the affinity which Penguins bear to Reptiles ... is shown in many parts of the structure, but a thorough examination of the chick in its progressive stages of growth *in ovo* cannot fail to throw a flood of light upon the ancestry and evolution of this very primitive type. It is from a thorough investigation of the Penguin and its life history that much light is expected to be thrown on the common origin and evolution of reptiles and birds'.[25]

ETW was reflecting an hypothesis proposed by Ernst Haeckel that ontogeny recapitulated phylogeny, that is, that the individual embryo of a developing organism passed through every stage of its species' evolution. It was also thought that the emperor penguin, belonging to one of the oldest known forms of fossil bird at that time, was a particularly primitive bird and that if there was a link between dinosaurs and birds it was most likely to be found, therefore, in the early embryonic stages of this species. Aligned with these ideas, Ted's aim was to make one of the biggest scientific breakthroughs of the twentieth century, by proving the link between dinosaurs and birds. Ted particularly wanted to find vestiges of teeth and to test theories connecting feathers with reptilian scales. The possibility of making this important scientific breakthrough therefore required visiting the emperor penguins soon after they had laid their eggs. On the previous *Discovery* expedition, Ted had concluded that emperor penguins must lay and incubate their eggs in the middle of the Antarctic winter, hence the need for a winter journey.

Just over three months after ETW's lecture, Ted selected two men, Henry 'Birdie' Bowers (1883-1912) and Apsley Cherry-Garrard (1886-1959),[26] to accompany him on the 130-mile trek from Cape Evans to Cape Crozier and back in the winter darkness. Against all the odds, in temperatures which sank as low as -60°C (-77°F), and amid raging blizzard conditions, in which even their tent was blown away, they survived the ordeal and succeeded in collecting three emperor penguin eggs. The achievement became immortalised in Cherry-Garrard's account of 'The Winter Journey', chapter seven of *The Worst Journey in the World* (1922). Later, although it was found that the eggs could not, in fact, prove any evolutionary connection between birds and dinosaurs, nevertheless, that very link was made in the 1990s based on the further embryology work of 'primitive' birds such as the ostrich. Therefore, Ted and ETW's original hypotheses were not that far off the mark.

What dangers Ted was experiencing in the Antarctic ETW could only imagine. During difficult times, ETW often drew comfort from his favourite trinity of Faith, Hope and Love. '*Hope* cheers, *Faith* strengthens, *Love* fulfils', he wrote, 'Each into each fresh power instils'.[27] On 5 October, it was faith that was required – though not for ETW - when he went to see his first aeroplane. The event was an exhibition flight given by Bentfield Charles Hucks (1884-1918) in a Blackburn monoplane with a 50-horse-power engine. ETW commented:

> Mr Hucks made a perfect ascent … and after a flight of half an hour or so alighted with admirable precision … the consummate management tended to minimise ones [sic] preconceived ideas of the danger and to give a confidence never felt before.[28]

While 'consummate management' safeguarded Hucks on this occasion, two days later, it was not enough: Hucks required an element of luck too when his petrol engine cut out whilst flying at a height of around 1,000 feet.[29] Perhaps luck was also to be needed in the Antarctic.

About a month later, ETW went to hear a lecture by Eric Marshall (1879-1963),[30] one of the members of Shackleton's *Nimrod* Expedition (1907–09). Although the slides were worn, ETW thought they were interesting, especially the ones of the penguins. More importantly, he commented, they 'enabled us to be with Ted in thought for a time and to realise the dangers he [was] facing'.[31] Two days later, ETW was able to feel tangibly closer to Ted, when he, Mary, Pollie and Ory went to London to see Herbert Ponting's films of the Antarctic, which were creating a sensation after release by the Gaumont Company. ETW commented:

... the [*Terra Nova*] cutting her way through the pack [ice], the huge ice cliffs of the barrier, and the moonlight views of Mts Erebus and Terror were extremely beautiful – while the ponies enjoying their freedom on landing from the Terra Nova, and the Adelie Penguins on the ice were wonderfully realistic. The whole gave an idea of Antarctic scenery and surroundings such as nothing else could have done.[32]

They returned to see the films two or three times more. Then, around New Year, while ETW was enjoying a 'very merry party'[33] with friends and relatives, Scott chose the final composition of the party to make the final journey of 169 miles to the Pole. In a decision that has been much criticised, Scott decided to take five men to the Pole rather than four: himself, Ted, Bowers, 'Titus' Oates and Petty Officer Evans. It meant a certain amount of re-organisation and whilst unplanned (all the supplies were packed in units of four) it was probably not as impulsive as some have suggested. However, the month of January proved to be a time of hardship, ill health and disappointment. At home, ETW was much saddened by the closure of the Jenner Society in Gloucester, following the death of Dr Francis Thomas Bond (1834-1911).[34] He worried that it now gave anti-vaccination campaigners free reign 'to say what they like without contradiction'.[35] By the end of the month, he was laid up in bed with flu and a temperature of 39°C (103°F). In the Antarctic, Ted was treating Evans's hand which had recently been cut and was full of pus. They were delayed by blizzards. As they hauled across the last miles to the Pole, they experienced a difficult surface for pulling. It was covered with ice crystals which clogged the sledge runners and slowed their nevertheless extraordinary progress. The temperatures which they faced on the Polar Plateau were also low, falling to -33°C (-27°F).

On 16 January, a short distance from the Pole, signs of Norwegian cairns, tracks and camps were seen. They were not, after all, to be the first to the South Pole. Amundsen, with his knowledge of Scott's plans ensured a head start, had travelled with dogs and encountering very little in the way of bad weather or delays had arrived five weeks before and was, in fact, almost back at his ship. Ted took the news with equanimity. Like his father, he thought that achievement of scientific discoveries was more important than worldly success.

They camped at the Pole on 17 January 1912. The wind was blowing at force four to six all day, in a temperature of -30°C (-22°F); Ted thought

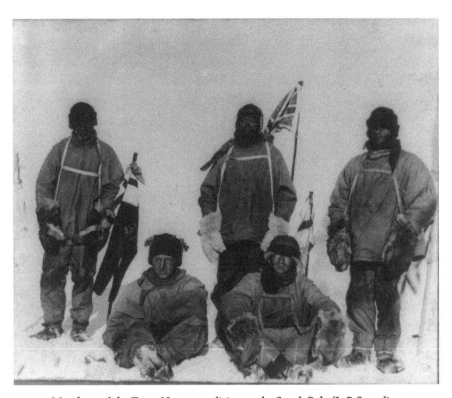

Members of the Terra Nova expedition at the South Pole (L-R Standing:
Robert F. Scott; Lawrence Oates; Henry R. Bowers; Seated: Ted; Edgar Evans.

it a 'very bitter day'.[36] With the wind chill it was unsurprising that Oates,
Evans and Bowers all suffered from 'pretty severe frost-bitten noses
and cheeks'.[37] On the following day, they took photographs and headed
north. The return journey now became a race to try to get back to the
ship before it departed again from the Antarctic. They started off well,
making good distances in low temperatures over difficult pulling surfaces
but, variously, started to suffer from frost-bite, snow blindness and falls
through tiredness.

On 9 February, as ETW was having a long talk with General Sir
Reginald Hart, (1848- 1931), the Irish British Army officer and recipient
of the Victoria Cross who was 'soon going out in Command to the Cape',[38]
Ted was taking a rest from marching through the snow to geologise
around the base of Mount Buckley, where Shackleton had found pieces
of coal. They collected 35 lbs of geological specimens in all, as they went
along the glacier, which were amongst the most important scientific

finds of the entire expedition. Although they were later criticised for not jettisoning the geological specimens when they got into difficulty, ETW, like Ted, recognised their potential importance to science. In a letter to the publisher Reginald Smith, ETW spoke excitedly about the 'precious rocks'[39] that Ted had collected. Previously, in 1902, ETW had observed:

A keen interest attaches to the finding of fossil remains on Antarctic land. Coal may be expected, and extinct forms nearly related to those of the Cretaceous and Early Tertiary formations. Palaeontology has not set foot on Antarctic soil, but it may yet find there a sphere of usefulness and absorbing interest.[40]

The fossils were later found to be the first Antarctic fossil specimens recorded by palaeobotanists of the genus *Glossopteris*, a type of fern, proving that the continent had once had a warm climate and providing a link to other continents in the Southern Hemisphere. This was crucial evidence for the Gondwana theory of continental origins, a scientific hypothesis that was emerging around this time. Coincidentally, during 1912, ETW presented specimens of Kenite, which Ted collected from Erebus Bay during a sledging trip in September 1902, to Cheltenham College Museum. ETW also donated other fossils and minerals to the museum in 1909 which were also collected by Ted.[41] Today, these valuable finds are held at The Wilson (Cheltenham Art Gallery and Museum).

The next day, following his conversation with Reginald Hart, ETW suffered from a severe relapse of influenza, coupled with a particularly persistent and troublesome cough, which kept him housebound for nearly a fortnight. In the Antarctic too, the five men started to suffer from 'persistent and troublesome' ailments and misfortune. Evans, who was visibly weakening, collapsed and died on 16 February. The remaining four continued but faced unusually low temperatures, often down to -40°C (-40°F), and, in a serious blow, found that each of their depots contained little oil, something they relied upon to melt drinking water and to cook.

The day after ETW recorded the birth of 'our Little Bettie',[42] his fifth grandchild and a new niece for Ted from his favourite sister Pollie, Ted stopped writing his diary. Then, 'during most of March', ETW wrote, 'I felt the effects of my illness and [was] not very fit for work of any kind'.[43] It was during this period that the final moments of the tragedy unfolded

in the Antarctic. On 2 March, as well as finding a shortage of oil at
another depot, Oates disclosed his blackened, frost-bitten feet. With cold
temperatures, fatigue, a bad pulling surface and either no wind or wind
from the north so that they could hoist no sail, it was clear that they were
in a serious position. His companions forced Ted to hand over the opium
tablets from the medical kit so that they could choose to end their lives,
if they so wished. Ted, in doing his best to nurse Oates, started to suffer
himself, getting more serious frostbite. They staggered on as best as they
could. Oates must have been in severe pain. On 16 or 17 March he could
take no more. In an effort to save his companions Oates walked out of the
tent and into a blizzard, famously saying 'I am just going outside and may
be some time'. Ted thought that Oates had shown very great courage in his
suffering and had died a noble death.

It was not enough. Scott, Ted and Bowers marched on for three
more days. Scott's feet were now badly frost-bitten, the best he could hope
for was amputation. They deposited some of their heavier equipment but
at Ted's special request continued to carry the geological specimens; 11
miles from the major supply cache at One Ton Depot they were again hit
by a blizzard. The three companions lay in their tent and finished their
fuel, whilst the blizzard raged around them. After laying up for a day or
two, Ted and Bowers intended to make a dash for supplies and to bring
food and fuel back to Scott. The weather never cleared enough for them to
attempt it. As the screaming blizzard raged outside, they decided to die a
natural death. They gradually starved and froze to death. Somehow, before
passing out, Ted found the strength to write some letters, including a last
one to his parents:

To Dr. E.T.Wilson
    Westal, Cheltenham

Dearest old Dad and Mother,
The end has come and with it an earnest looking forward to the day when
we shall all meet together in the hereafter. Death has no terrors for me. I
am only sorry for my beloved Ory and for all of you dear people, but it is
God's will and all is for the best. Our record is clear and we have struggled
against very heavy odds to the bitter end – two of the 5 of us are already
dead and we three are nearly done up. Scott's foot is badly frostbitten so

that he can scarcely walk. Dear old home folks how I love you all and how I have loved to think of you all – bless you. I have had a very happy life and I look forward to a very happy life hereafter when we shall all be together again. God knows I have no fear in meeting Him – for He will be merciful to all of us. My poor Ory may or may not have long to wait – I am so sorry for her. However we have done all for the best believing in His guidance and we have both believed that whatever is, is His will, and in that faith I am prepared to meet Him and leave all you loved ones in His care till His own time is fulfilled.

     Now God be with you all,

     Your own loving Ted[44]

The letter was written about 21 or 22 March 1912. Back in Cheltenham the family was blissfully unaware of the tragedy that had unfolded in the Antarctic. On 3 April they received the 'Last News from South Pole Plateau' from Ory whose telegram from New Zealand reported 'Ted absolutely fit exceedingly happy.'[45] On the following day the *Cheltenham Examiner* explained how 'the party of heroes' were within 150 miles[46] of the Pole on 3 January, Captain Scott having sent Lieutenant Evans and three men back with the message that was subsequently published through the Central News Agency. Whether or not they would succeed would not be known for twelve months, but as the *Examiner* concluded, '...in Capt. Scott's own words, "the prospect of success [for the five, including 'the son of Dr E.T. Wilson'] seemed good"'.[47]

On 17 April, ETW took photographs of the solar eclipse, the results of which, he thought, resembled 'illuminated kidney beans'.[48] He was also busy contributing to work on the flints of the Cotswolds that his friend George B. Witts (1846-1912),[49] an authority on the subject, had started. In June, he shared in Ted's excitement following the success of the Cape Crozier expedition through writing to Reginald Smith. Describing the three emperor penguin eggs that Ted had collected as 'a veritable treasure', he thought that their subsequent analysis would repay the dangers involved in the hazardous journey.[50] In July, as CNSS President, ETW continued his own local scientific exploration by leading a 3-mile walk from Coombe Hill, one of Ted's favourite places for exploring wildlife, to Wainlode. Despite unfavourable conditions, a wealth of botanical specimens was identified.[51]

In August, ETW and Mary travelled to London where, with Pollie and her husband Godfrey, they saw another selection of Ponting's 3,000 feet worth of film shot during the earlier parts of the *Terra Nova* expedition. Commenting about the screening, put on by the Gaumont Company at the Palace Theatre, the *Pall Mall Gazette* remarked:

> Notoriously we are a phlegmatic people, but there must have been few who could watch without a strange kind of emotion such pictures as the cinematograph then threw upon the screen for the first time.[52]

For ETW, it was the tent scene that, in retrospect, seemed 'a cruel mockery'.[53] For this, Ted, Scott, Bowers and Evans 'went through all the stages of camp doings in the tent',[54] from changing their footgear, hanging up their socks, and cooking their food, to unrolling their sleeping bags and getting ready for bed.

Less than three months later, on 12 November 1912, as yet still unknown to the family, a search party led by the expedition Surgeon, Dr Atkinson, discovered the bodies of Ted, Scott and Bowers in the tent. All the members of the party were deeply moved by what they saw: Ted, half reclining and sitting facing the door of the tent wrapped in his sleeping bag, his arms crossed over his chest, with a gentle smile on his face, looking for all the world as if he was about to wake up; Bowers toggled up in his bag; and Scott, lying with his arm thrust out of his bag towards Ted. Their bodies showed signs of their ordeal. After a brief examination, their diaries, personal belongings and the geological specimens were collected. Atkinson read the burial service; they sang *Onward Christian Soldiers* and collapsed the tent over them as they lay. Above them they built a great cairn of snow surmounted with a cross of skis and they were left to lie in the peace of the Antarctic. The bodies of Oates and Evans were never found. On Observation Hill a wooden memorial cross was erected looking out over the Great Ice Barrier, now the tomb in which their bodies would drift slowly towards the sea. With their names, at Cherry-Garrard's suggestion, the closing line from Tennyson's *Ulysses* was carved: 'To strive, to seek, to find and not to yield'.

Back at home, the obsession with all things Antarctic continued apace. The family was either busy admiring Ted's sketches that had been sent back with the relief ship or debating whether to go and listen to a triumphant Amundsen, who was already engaged in a major lecture tour.

He came to Cheltenham on 30 November, when he gave two lectures 'in an unaffected and straightforward fashion' at the Town Hall, vividly describing, as the *Cheltenham Looker-On* put it, 'the difficulties, the perils, the pleasures and the success of the Expedition ... from the fitting up of the *Fram* to the planting of the Norwegian flag at the South Pole....[55] Five days earlier, ETW had gone again to see Ponting's pictures. He lingered at the ones of Ted, gazing at those of him 'smiling there in the tent and holding his pony', later recalling that Ted had been lying 'in his frozen tomb' since March 'after one of the most heroic struggles ever recorded – a life laid down for his friends'.[56] As a photographer himself ETW greatly admired Ponting's work not just because of their technical brilliance but also because of the difficult circumstances under which they were produced. He commented:

> Every drop of water has to be produced from frozen snow, and developing carried on at night when non-photographers were snoozing in their bunks.[57]

Around this time, ETW was also preoccupied with giving a (repeated) lecture on the 'Flora and Fauna of Great Britain and Ireland'[58] to the Field Club at Dean Close. By applying Darwinian environmental principles ETW explained some of the mysteries relating to our native wildlife: why three species of freshwater herring are only found in the lakes of southwest Scotland, northwest England, Wales and Ireland; why there are no snakes in Ireland; and why some species have survived whilst others have died out. Towards the end of the lecture he referred to Ted's discovery at *The Crippetts* of the fact that pygmy shrews would be unable to thrive if faced by competition from the field mouse and the common shrew.[59]

It would still be more than two months before ETW, now eighty years old, would learn the tragic news that the Polar party had not survived their final ordeal. The first that the family at *Westal* knew that something was not right was the receipt of a telegram on 10 February 1913 saying that the expedition had returned early due to disaster but to hope for the best. ETW recalled:

> The staggering blow came on the evening of Feb. 10th; I had been at a meeting of the Delancey [Hospital] Trustees and during the whole time

had been perturbed by the news that the *Terra Nova* had arrived in New Zealand. As she was before her time, I anticipated bad news and in the evening a telegram came from May Wilson giving no particulars but sympathising with us and hoping the news was not true. Then ensued a period of suspense almost unbearable – until the truth burst upon us in all its terrible reality – the hopes of years in a moment dashed to the ground. No words can explain what our dear Ted meant to us all and to our dear, good Ory, vainly awaiting his return in New Zealand. It was a sad, sad time.[60]

The impact of the news of the death of Scott and his party has largely been forgotten today. The closest contemporary event for comparison would be the death of Diana, Princess of Wales. There was an international media frenzy which helped to build a myth. This image of Scott and his companions as heroes has been extensively criticised, but the commentators rather miss the point. The perception of a hero as someone who is perfect is as false as the modern notion of a saint. The concepts of heroism which resonated as the news broke were much older ones. Classical epic heroes often die at the peak of their worldly achievement, they die well, and they die due to their human flaws. To a classically educated generation, such heroes were Scott and his companions - a much richer and deeper concept of heroism which allows them their humanity. In this sense it was not false for the Cheltenham papers to hail Ted as 'Cheltenham's Antarctic Hero', dying an heroic and noble death in the service of his country, like Scott, Bowers, Evans and Oates. In this sense, a similar 'heroic and noble death' was endured by General Gordon at Khartoum. The entire family was plunged into grief. ETW recalled:

Sympathy poured in on every side from relations and friends, some of them unheard of for years, from acquaintances and perfect strangers. It was a help but nought could soothe the aching heart – and it was long before the realisation of the noble self-sacrifice and devotion to Duty even unto death began to take the place of our own selfish grief. Like our dear Nell, our Saintly Ted had given his life for his friends – and a whole nation mourned the loss of these noble lives.[61]

Across the nation and the empire, memorial services were held. The family was too upset to attend the national memorial service attended by the King at St Paul's Cathedral on 14 February, where more than 10,000 people stood outside unable to get in. They held instead 'a quiet little service of [their] own at home'.[62] In Cheltenham, there were well attended memorial services in St Matthew's Church and in the Cheltenham College Chapel where ETW thought that '[Canon] Waterfield's address was touching as well as truly appreciative'.[63] One of the many services held in Gloucestershire made national headlines when it was reported that the vicar of Cam Parish Church, the Revd Griffiths, died in his pulpit after referring to the death of Captain Scott and his party.

Letters of condolence and telegrams of sympathy continued to flood into *Westal*. Much of the spotlight fell on ETW given his popularity and high profile throughout the town. As a result of this, glowing tributes were paid not only to Ted but also to his father in direct appreciation of the indefatigable work he had provided to the community. Some of the tributes came from organisations and institutions for which ETW had done much invaluable work. A typical example came from the Cotswold Convalescent Home. The report from the meeting stated:

> [They] deeply sympathised with [ETW] in the great loss he had sustained, but could not help thinking that the consolation must be equal to the sorrow, for to feel himself in the honoured position of being the father of such a son, or to have a knowledge of the splendid work that son had done, and to think that he had had the bringing up of that son, and that he had taken a line in the world, the line of science so near his father's heart, and so distinguished himself, must indeed be a great honour to any man.[64]

ETW thought that the insensitive reporting in certain quarters of such an intimate moment of their lives was deeply hurtful. He became particularly upset when some suggested that the bodies should be brought home, and so he wrote to the publisher Reginald Smith (of Smith, Elder and Co.), urging him to stop this proposal.[65] On 19 February, a letter in *The Times* appeared from 'a near relative' signed W (but believed to be ETW),[66] imploring that the bodies should not be transported to New Zealand or home for burial. It urged:

Let them sleep on amid the eternal snows, the scene of their great
achievement, and beneath the cairn which the loving hearts and hands of
their comrades have erected to their memory.[67]

Whilst Ted's body was left to lie in peace in the Antarctic, a simple
inscription was later added to his parent's gravestone in St Peter's church
graveyard, Leckhampton. It recorded the death of Ted 'who died with
Captain Scott after reaching the South Pole 12th March 1912'[68] alongside
his mother whose epitaph reads 'She loved much' and his father, of whom
it said that 'He went about doing good'.

A fortnight after the 'staggering blow' from the Antarctic, further
bad news arrived. 'Alas! Misfortunes seldom come singly',[69] noted ETW.
On 24 February, Ted's younger brother Jim was instructed to take 'an
absolute and prolonged rest of at least 6 months'[70] due to overwork
amid difficult circumstances at his new vicarage of St Andrew's Church at
Wolverhampton. Previously, ETW and Mary had endured the tragic loss of
three children, Nellie, Jessica and Gwladys. The number of deaths was not
an unusual occurrence in large Victorian families of the time. However,
the huge outpouring of grief and media frenzy surrounding the tragedy of
Scott's party made it particularly difficult to cope with Ted's death.

In Cheltenham, shocked by the heroic loss of one of its own, the
mayor sought permission from ETW for arrangements to be made for
an appropriate memorial. 'At first Dr. Wilson', the Cheltenham Examiner
reported, 'with the delicacy which those who are acquainted with him
recognise as characteristic, was reluctant to receive a memorial'. However,
after being given assurances 'that such would be the wish of the town, he
agreed to the proposal, merely suggesting, very naturally, that the family
might be consulted as to the form the memorial might take'.[71] Like his
father, Ted would not have accepted easily the idea of a memorial. Medals
and statues would have flattered Ted - overwhelmed him even - but not
impressed him. While some clamoured for a Wilson gallery in Cheltenham,
adorned with 'a sculptured copy of a sledge drawn by a full team of
Esquimaux dogs, and accompanied by ski-shod explorers'[72] and penguin
columns, ETW's initial suggestion was for 'a memorial connected with the
General Hospital ...'.[73] Later, he recommended a bronze statue that could
be sculptured by Kathleen Scott (Scott's widow).[74] The discussion also
presented an opportunity for the Town Council to express appreciation

for ETW's indefatigable work for Cheltenham: the Mayor noted that 'there has never been any movement mooted for the advantage of our town of which he [ETW] has not been a prominent and active supporter', while Alderman Winterbotham spoke about him as 'always [having] been foremost in anything that has affected the welfare or benefit of the town'.[75] A public subscription list was opened to raise the necessary funds. About 400 subscribers were obtained, but in the end a reduced fee was agreed with Lady Scott.[76]

While the plans for a public memorial progressed, ETW was inspired during April to write two personal tributes for Ted in verse. They helped him to come to terms with his grief, made worse through the absence of a body which could be buried in the family graveyard. The first, composed around the time ETW eagerly awaited the return of the nightingale's song, was entitled 'The Crippetts. In Memoriam "Ted"'.[77]

Hark to the songsters in yon flowery grove!
That grove now sacred, to his memory dear.
Where not in rapture he was wont to rove
And note the changes of the opening year.
For him the tiny disclosed her nest,
Her sweetest notes for him the Mavis trilled,
The Warblers' song his very soul possessed
And stirred the deeps, with vibrant music thrilled.
The flush of early dawn, the sunset glow
The subtle tints half sun on bush or tree,
Revealed to him what few but he might know
And gave him freely of their mystery.
Now he knows all – and with unclouded eye
Reads the full wonders of the sea and sky.
The birds sing on – and who shall I dare to say
He hears them now where breaks the eternal day.

The second poem, which incorporated quotations from the journals of *Scott's Last Expedition* (1913) and the journals of Tryggve Gran (1888-1980), a member of the search party that discovered the frozen bodies on 12 November 1912, was entitled 'Contrasts in Antarctica'.[78]

The Tempest raged – in elemental Strife
The Blizzard shrieked and howled – and Lo!
A solitary tent; - (no sign of life;)
Lay buried deep in drifts of blinding Snow.
Within - was hallowed peace - Three lay at rest,
One smiling gazed with hopefull (*sic*) calm blue eyes;
The Leader leaning on a comrades (*sic*) breast,
Had penned glad tribute to their memories.
"Death held no terrors" for they gave their all,
(Leaving rough notes the heroic tale to tell)
And died unwavering at the Masters (*sic*) call
For Honour, Country, Comrades - "All is well",
Let them sleep on beneath the Cairn of Snow
(What nobler Monument could Earth bestow?)
Let them sleep on; no fitter resting place
For Heroes, worthy of their (the all conquering) Warrior race.[79]

Ory arrived back in England in April 1913, having sailed home accompanied by Dr Atkinson and her sister, Constance. She went to live at *Westal* for some time. Once back in England many expedition members came to call at *Westal* and several, including Frank Debenham[80] and Apsley Cherry-Garrard, were regular visitors. Dr Atkinson[81] reported privately on the finding of the bodies and stated categorically that there was no trace of scurvy (often incorrectly suggested as the cause of their deaths) to be seen on the bodies - scurvy was probably incipient and a contributory factor amongst many others. Lieutenant (now Commander) Evans lectured across the country on the expedition to packed houses, speaking in Cheltenham on 14 November 1913, when he also stayed at *Westal*.

Apart from supporting each other through the loss of their son, ETW and Mary also did their best to support the grieving mothers of Ted's fellow Antarctic explorers. In June, Emily Bowers, née Webb, mother of 'Birdie', visited *Westal*. ETW commented, 'she poor woman mourns an only son – a treasure of great price – and one of the mainstays of the S. Polar sledging party'.[82] A year later, still haunted by her son's self-sacrifice, Caroline Oates, called at *Westal*. What words of comfort ETW, Mary and Ory offered her were not recorded but the fact that Ted had written to her that, 'He died like a man and a soldier, without a word of regret or complaint'[83] may have provided some solace.

In July, ETW and Mary were cheered by a visit from Ted's comrades from the *Terra Nova*, the geologist Raymond Priestley (1886-1974), who donated some minerals collected during Shackleton's *Nimrod* Expedition, and the geographer Thomas Griffith Taylor (1880-1964). ETW recorded:

> ...[they] were loud in their praises of Ted, Uncle Bill, the Peacemaker and trusted advisor in all cases of difficulty and doubt. Griffith Taylor an Australian, rough and unkempt but of true metal – clever, witty and a true man – Priestley more stolid but true as steel and to be utterly trusted under any conditions.[84]

As the summer drew to a close, ETW noted sadly about the lack of financial support being given to the Delancey Hospital.[85] In October this necessitated transfer of its control to a Board of Management governed by the Cheltenham Corporation, the Cheltenham Rural District Council, and the Charlton Kings District Council.[86] For ETW, now in his eightieth year, it was the end of an association that had lasted forty-two years, and, bitterly, he reflected how the hospital had now been 'thrown to the wolves'.[87]

In October, while still presiding as CNSS President, he gave a paper on 'The Long-Barrow Men of the Cotswolds'. In it, partly paying tribute to his old friend, the archaeologist George B. Witts (1846-1912), ETW stressed the importance of employing proper scientific methods given that eighteen of the forty long barrows in Gloucestershire had been examined in an amateurish manner and much useful evidence had been 'unrecorded or lost'.[88] To illustrate this, he recounted the following story:

> ... an enterprising dentist [found] a Neolithic skull convenient for practising his art, [but] at the whisper of an accusing conscience, restored it to its original burial-place provided with gold stopping up-to-date.[89]

If ever there was a time to re-establish proper rigour in scientific methodology it was now. Around three months later, ETW was shown the Piltdown skull[90] by Dr Arthur Smith Woodward (1864-1944) who, as the then Keeper of Geology at the Natural History Museum, had worked with the amateur archaeologist Charles Dawson (1864-1916) on the various finds near the Sussex village of Piltdown. Then claimed to be the 'missing link' between ape and man, it was not until 1949 that the extent of the audacious hoax was revealed.[91]

ETW never recovered from the tragic loss of Ted. At the beginning of 1914 he commented, 'My health was now thoroughly broken and my walking powers reduced to a variable quantity'.[92] He was suffering from fibrositis (now known as fibromyalgia), which is often brought on by a traumatic bereavement. It seems possible that the condition was triggered by Ted's death and the associated media frenzy. Despite this, he was able to summon up sufficient energy to show Henry Balfour (1863-1939), the first curator of the Pitt Rivers Museum, the recently-added collection of flints at the Cheltenham museum and, a fortnight later, to see Ted's pictures, which were now exhibiting in the local art gallery.[93] Yet, in March, after consulting Sir William Osler about some recent attacks of fibrositis, which

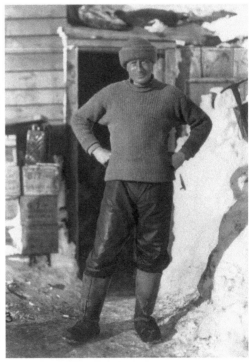

were weakening his muscles, he was pronounced 'absolutely sound' and told that he should live until 100.[94]

By early summer, final preparations were being made for the unveiling of Ted's statue by Sir Clements Markham on the Promenade on 9 July. On the day itself, ETW, Mary and Ory attended a luncheon hosted by the mayor at the Town Hall. Afterwards, they formed part of the group that sat on a raised platform in front of the statue. The only decorative colour was provided by a large Union Jack that fluttered gently. Before the ceremony began, the band of the 5th Gloucesters played patriotic

Ted in Antarctica, 1911. This characteristic pose was later used by Lady Scott for his statue.

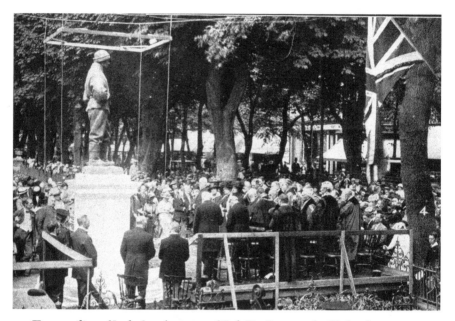

The unveiling of Lady Scott's statue of Ted, The Promenade, Cheltenham 1914

songs, including *Land of Hope and Glory*. ETW had already seen Lady Scott's design of the statue during a visit to London,[95] which showed Ted in characteristic pose, standing with right hand poised on hip. She used one of Ponting's photographs as a reference for this, and supplemented it with Apsley Cherry-Garrard who acted as a model, wearing corduroy trousers. When the statue, cast in very dark bronze, was unveiled a loud cheer went up; because the sun was shining behind the statue, the crowd

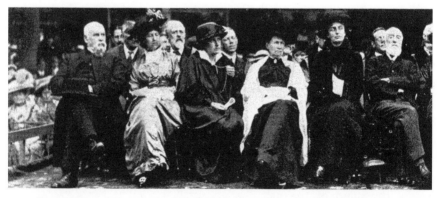

Part of the group on the raised platform. Front Row: L-R Rev. Souper; Miss Skillicorne; Lady Scott; Mary Agnes Wilson; Oriana Wilson; ETW.

in front could not immediately appreciate its fine craftsmanship and detail. Nevertheless, Louis Bernacchi (1876-1942), a close friend of Ted's and chief physicist on the *Discovery* expedition, was one of many who commented on 'the characteristic likeness of the statue'.[96]

ETW remarked, 'Sir Clements spoke very well and feelingly of Ted and Lady Scott was able to see how much her work was appreciated'.[97] ETW was also grateful to the local MP, James T. Agg-Gardner (1846-1928), for paying tribute to ETW's friend, the late James Winterbotham[98] at the ceremony. Afterwards, there was a large private reception at *Westal* which greatly sapped ETW's energy.[99] Physical pain ensued. Five days later, ETW wrote to Apsley Cherry-Garrard, apologising for his scrawl, due to being laid up in bed on his back after an attack of fibrositis.[100] He regretted the lack of an opportunity for a 'quiet chat' during the unveiling of the statue, but thanked him for 'taking part with us in our pride and in our sorrow'.[101] Worse 'pain' was about to follow.

19
War and Death (1914-18)

First World War – ETW's worsening illness – Infectious diseases –
Bernard's active service – Sir William Osler – Antarctic portrait of Ted – A
Retrospect – Golden wedding anniversary – Death

'Dare we venture to hope that peace not war, love not hate, may be the key note
of the coming century?'
~ ETW ~

WHEN BRITAIN ENTERED THE First World War on 4 August 1914
it was with an overriding sense of relief 'after the shilly shallying
of our invertebrate Government'[1] that ETW recorded this decision in his
journal. While the news still came as a shock, his observation perhaps
reflects the later assertion of the Foreign Secretary, Edward Grey, and the
Chancellor, Lloyd George, that the Cabinet's decision was fully justified on
the basis of the public mood at the time, as expressed through widespread
demonstrations in favour of war, even though the Government was still
pondering the alternative of peace.[2]

A fortnight later, ETW received the first of many letters from
Bernard who had volunteered, despite being over the accepted age of
forty-one. Prior to being gazetted Captain in the 6th King's Own Yorkshire
Light Infantry in September, he was busy buying horses: 'I hope [they] will
be my last', he commented from Doncaster, 'as it is a sad business'.[3] In
total he bought seventy-five, two-thirds of which were mares, at a cost of
£3,172. Ironically, all the geldings had been sold and exported to Germany
and Russia. While no-one could have predicted the estimated eight million
horses[4] which were to be slaughtered on the battle fields, ETW was under
no illusion about human beings' destructive capability, acquired in part by
his 'planning brain [which] at once raised him above the law of the jungle'.[5]
In a rather prophetic lecture given in 1898 to the CNSS, he commented:

> ...man has never scrupled to kill his fellow man... [...]. The best intellects,
> the best workmen are engaged in preparations for war; millions of men,

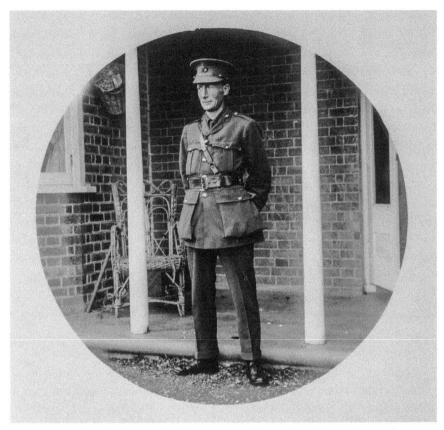

Bernard in Copthorne after being gazetted Captain, 23 September 1914

many of them the very flower of their several nations, ready at the word of command to fling themselves into a conflict in which they may have little or no personal concern ... [...] New rifle is followed by new rifle, new bullet by one more murderous than the last; machine guns and smokeless powder, explosives of ever increasing power, nation trying to outdo nation in the ingenuity and destructiveness of its equipment.[6]

Looking back to events that had been developing since 1859, ETW commented on the absurd arms race that was taking place between Europe's six major powers. The scale was disturbing: 17 million people involved in fighting; 10 million more, directly or indirectly employed in supporting roles for warfare; and as much as £1 million spent on a single battleship and £20,000 on a 110-ton gun. 'How is it all to end?' he asked, 'and to what goal are we tending? Are the civilised nations to grapple in a Titanic conflict, leaving a hecatomb of dead and a sad legacy of crippled lives?'[7]

As war at the Western Front intensified, so did ETW's physical pain. Despite a short period of 'quiescence and improvement', his weight dropped well below 9 stone.[8] In October, his doctor tried a vaccine to alleviate his suffering, but with limited success. Just as a lull in the fighting in the Flanders trenches seemed to initially raise hopes and expectations that the war would be over by Christmas, only to be dashed by an ever-greater number of casualties, so the injections into ETW's frail body led to more acute attacks after a short period of respite. Then followed a growing realisation that his body was incapable of producing sufficient antibodies, and so just as Tommy would have to accept that he would not be home by Christmas, so ETW was forced to succumb to a continuing long-term pain. Greatly concerned, Bernard wrote:

> Dear old Dad. You must stick it out to see the end of the war. We shall soon be very near the border line of this world and the next. - You dear old man will, it seems, have to suffer as much as any of us, who go to the front. [...] If I have to leave you – you must live on for the family and then on the other side – what a happy family we shall be to meet you and the old mother – Ted and Neli Gladdie and Jessie – we shall give you a great welcome.[9]

It was not just the military threats that endangered Bernard's life. When not focusing on his own pain, ETW was acutely aware of the threats posed by his son's potential exposure to infectious diseases. Previously, he had written:

> The microbe is now the most active and formidable of the enemies of the human race, and the survival of the fittest will not necessarily be to the strong in mind or body, but to such as are more immune, whether by nature or by art, to such diseases as smallpox, scarlet fever, measles, typhoid, diphtheria, and tuberculosis.[10]

During the First and Second Boer Wars (1880-81, 1899-1902) in South Africa two-thirds of all British deaths had been accounted for

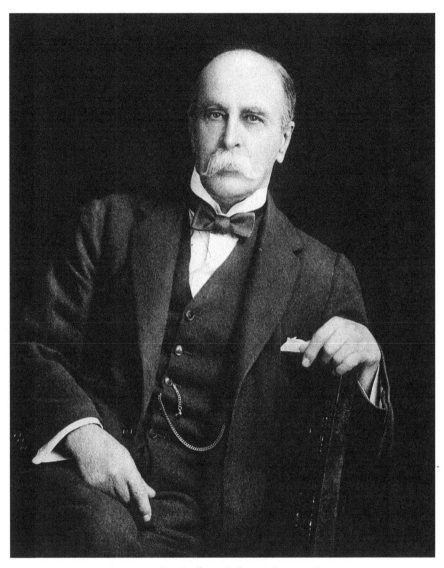

Portrait of Sir William Osler, at the age of 70.

through disease; therefore, it was clear that 'the Germans were not the
only enemy'.[11] Microbes were potentially more insidious foes. In October,
ETW initially became anxious when Bernard, then stationed with his
company at Aldershot, reported a diphtheria case.[12] If only ETW could
have overseen the management of the disease, yet he was too weak and
confined to his bed to be able to offer much more than loving thoughts

and prayers. As far as typhoid was concerned, however, ETW had his 'genial and true'[13] friend, Sir William Osler, Regius Professor of Medicine at the University of Oxford, to thank for ensuring that troops were adequately protected through vaccination. Osler, whom ETW befriended during his organising role for the 1901 BMA conference in Cheltenham, had been successful in persuading senior army officers of the need to vaccinate troops against the disease; this was despite strong lobbying from anti-vaccination campaigners and a conscientious objector law which prevented compulsory vaccination.[14] Cholera was another significant concern. For this, Bernard took the precaution of asking his mother to make him two cholera belts[15] of thin white flannel which he thought should afford good protection.

By the time ETW celebrated his eighty-second birthday, the impending danger to his son, who was about to cross the Channel and go out to the Western Front, suddenly hit home. Anticipating that his father would remain healthy and able to live for another ten years, Bernard hoped that, once he returned home, they would be able to enjoy a day of fishing or hunting together. He wrote to his father:

> You know I love you very very dearly ... I hope to see you again somehow – either at Godalming[16] or London if you can get strong enough before I go abroad. But if we don't well – we know each other well enough and love each other well enough to bear up and be cheery even if we don't meet up again before I go out.[17]

Nevertheless, from early 1915, ETW had become increasingly house-bound, and started to feel increasingly frustrated that he was unable to attend events and meetings or contribute to public work. Bernard was equally frustrated: keen to contribute directly to the fighting as soon as possible, he was losing patience as his deployment orders continued to be delayed. ETW was relieved that Bernard, at least for the time being, remained on home soil. In February, he heard from Pollie, writing from Bushey. While she spoke about an injured soldier who had just returned from action after killing forty Germans, her letter also brought with it the hope that the war might be over by May if Germany were to be 'driven to peace by want of metal and hunger'.[18]

Bernard continued to worry about his father's physical health, but was pleasantly surprised to see him looking well after paying a flying visit

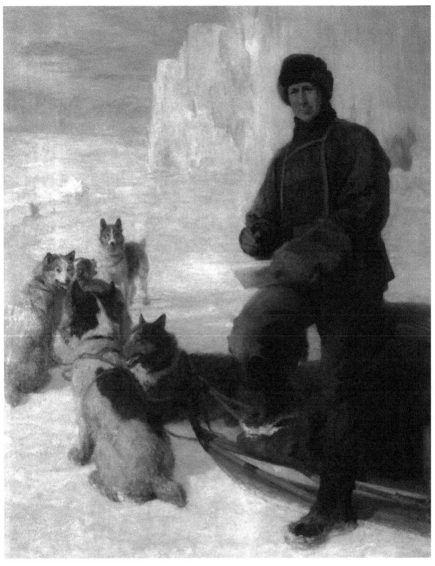

Portrait of Dr E. A. Wilson by J. Briton Rivière (1915).

home from Brocton Camp, on Cannock Chase: 'I was afraid he was more
pulled down than he is', he wrote to his mother. 'Oh! He will buck up with
the summer and be out walking on Cleeve Hill – pray God!'[19] In March,
ETW's spirits were temporarily lifted by news that an above-life-size
portrait of Ted had just been completed by Briton Rivière.[20] Commissioned
by Cheltenham College the painting was produced posthumously from

historic photographs. However, his joy was tinged with sadness when he realised that he would probably never see it, other than through a photograph.

Unable to leave *Westal*, ETW's social life relied on visits from family and friends. It was equally upsetting for ETW and his grandchildren when they found him lying in bed, his 'white beard draping over the toes'.[21] While he was too tired and sick to speak very much, they greatly treasured the letters they received from him, richly illustrated with tiny pen and ink drawings. Among the many well-wishers was Sir William Osler, who visited in June. Still working as Regius Chair of Medicine at Oxford, at the time the most prestigious medical appointment in the English-speaking world, Osler was flat out dealing with the most challenging cases from the hundreds of wounded soldiers returning to British hospitals.[22] Nevertheless, he found time to 'snatch a brief bookman's holiday'[23] when he lunched at Cheltenham Ladies' College, and visited the extensive manuscripts collection in Sir Thomas Phillipps' library at Thirlestaine House.[24] It is likely that it was during this trip that Osler included a short visit to his dear, old friend. Osler would have been saddened to see ETW's gaunt figure, his weight having dropped to just 8 stone. On this occasion, ETW probably gave Osler the detailed records he kept of his symptoms from May 1913 to 26 April 1916, about which Osler commented:

> Remarkable case, remarkable record, and a remarkable old man; a fine type of the English naturalist-physician and of the cultivated provincial consultant. [...] The case itself is a very unusual one – a fibrositis, with nodules, chiefly of the adductor muscles.[25]

While ETW's strength hit rock bottom, a devastating telegram arrived on 20 July, informing the family that Bernard had been wounded. He was subsequently invalided to a hospital at Woolwich where he received treatment for a head wound. Later, ETW became irate after Bernard, who continued to suffer from severe headaches, was discharged prematurely and sent back for duty to Rugby. At least, for the time being, Bernard was spared frontline duty; and, by the end of the year, his training and administrative skills had been so highly prized that he was appointed Chief Entrenchment Officer to one of the Divisions at Stafford – an important post entailing responsibility for the teaching of 30,000 recruits, including officers.

In October 1915, as ETW was approaching his eighty-third birthday, he felt compelled to take a comprehensive look back over his life and review his successes and failures. He called it 'A Retrospect'. It was originally intended to be read only by members of his family.[26] Although only seven pages long, it comes as a surprise to the reader, coming as it does after two large volumes of rich, life-affirming memories. In this scathing self-analysis he berates himself for having made several major mistakes. He is emphatic, for example, given his time again, that he would have done things differently. On a professional level he would have avoided coming to Cheltenham, but would have lived somewhere with a well-respected medical school, probably Liverpool or Oxford (where he was once offered a post at the Radcliffe Royal Infirmary), but not London for he 'loathed London and London life'.[27] Instead, his happy marriage and the birth of ten children had led him to put down deep roots in Cheltenham.

Weighing up his strengths and weaknesses, he recognised that, had he joined the army, as his brother Charly had done, he would have made an excellent subordinate officer, largely by dint of his willingness to work hard and not shirk responsibility. However, he added, 'God help the army that I was ever called upon to command'.[28] Rather poignantly, he felt the absence of some kind of mentor, 'someone to guide and advise but there was no one, no one at School no one at Oxford no one at the Hospital no one in Cheltenham'.[29] It seems likely that these harsh comments arose partly through the effects of his illness, including the possibility that he may have then also been suffering from depression, and partly through a sense of being overshadowed by the success of Charly and the fame of Ted, whose loss he felt so acutely.

In spite of having just penned 'A Retrospect' at the end of October, ETW enjoyed a remarkable short period of good health - so much so that he felt well enough to visit Cheltenham College to see Rivière's portrait of Ted. Anticipating how much he would admire the portrait, following the unveiling ceremony that had taken place in the College library[30] on 18 September, which Mary attended in his absence, ETW was moved to tears. The magnificent portrait showed Ted standing in polar dress against a sledge with a distant view of Mount Erebus in the background. It proved to be the family's favourite memorial to Ted, although Bernard did not fully approve of it.[31] ETW also saw the brass memorial of Ted bearing the Wilson crest and motto that had been placed behind the choir on the north side of the chapel, in a stall where ETW had regularly worshipped. In the adjoining stall was a similar brass, commemorating Charly. Here together were two celebrated figures of the British Empire, both high-profile explorers and revered Old Cheltonians - perhaps the two most remarkable members of the Wilson family to date.

It was around this time that ETW put down in words his idea of heaven as far as he could conceive it: 'it would be at all events spiritual', he thought, 'freed from all idea of corporeal or material existence ...'.[32] Drawing on his love for nature, he likened it to the image of a dragonfly that was creeping in the mud and unable to conceive of 'the glorious future before it of basking in the sunshine and freedom of flight'.[33] While he looked forward to entering heaven, the memories of his heroic son and brother probably weighed heavily on his mind.

For ETW, it was the definite end of an era when, on 16 December, the Delancey Trust was finally wound up and the building handed over to the new governing body. 'May our successors meet with equal good fortune in the control of infection and the treatment of disease,' he commented, 'and live up to the ideal which for so many years had been set before them'.[34] From 1948, the Delancey Hospital was converted into an elderly care

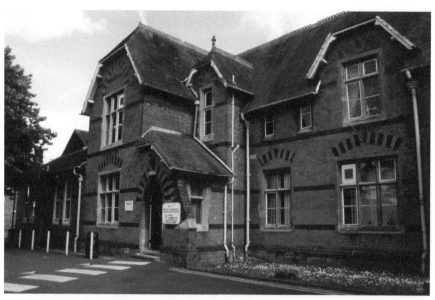

Delancey Hospital shortly before it was developed for residential use.

hospital and, in 2013, the buildings converted into apartments and the grounds developed for further residential use.

Any sadness that ETW still felt about this was soon replaced by the excitement that Bernard could come home for Christmas. He was so buoyed up by his son's visit that he summoned up sufficient energy to carve the turkey, and he penned a short poem to mark the occasion, adding the following accompanying remarks: 'Grant our brave ones victory' and 'Bring universal peace'.[35] Among the gallant officers fighting at the Front were Charles and Francis, ETW's two nephews, whose progress he had followed since the Boer Wars. While they continued to win medals and mentions in despatches, by the close of the year their great uncle's frailty returned. From then on, ETW ceased writing his journal.

As the war dragged on, again there was renewed hope that it may be over 'by next winter'.[36] Yet, there were also the worrying new developments in tank and chemical warfare. There was now a growing sense of truth in ETW's remark that nations in war compete 'in the ingenuity and destructiveness of [their] equipment'.[37] In February, Bernard wrote to his father from Brocton Camp about his contribution to an experiment aimed at discovering the impact of a British gas cylinder being accidentally blown up by enemy shells dropping into British trenches.[38] The purpose was to test the strength and density of the gas in the trench compared with a distance of 30 feet away. Although no casualties were suffered during the controlled experiment, the risks were all too apparent. Bernard wrote:

The gas was very visible in bulk but invisible though deadly in the trench – one part in 10,000 [proving] fatal.[39]

At the beginning of February, ETW suffered another acute attack of fibrositis. Hoping to present a paper on Ted's expedition to Cape Crozier for the Friends in Council, he was laid up in bed at *Westal* as his paper was read by the FiC secretary.[40] Lacking the opportunity to see ETW at first hand, Bernard monitored his father's health through the firmness of his script, as revealed through letters sent from home. Once, after receiving ETW's comments on some of his draft lecture notes, he became concerned that his father's writing had become 'very stiff'.[41] Bernard also became increasingly concerned about his father's weight, prompting him to advise his father that 'an oyster or two' was not enough to keep up his strength.[42]

Record of ETW's paper from the Friends in Council Minutes Book,
1 February 1916.

By March 1916, at Brocton Camp, Bernard discovered that Antarctic conditions had suddenly arrived. The ground 'crevassed quite over with no indication of a six foot trench under the snow'.[43] As he walked out for about 100 yards, the snow well above his knees while thinking about the feasibility of the French beating off the German advance on Verdun, he drew inspiration from Ted. He wrote:

...he is a brother to have been proud of and an example to follow. I trust I shall be given courage and strength of character to face danger when my time comes'.[44]

Next month Bernard braced himself for perhaps the biggest challenge in his life as he prepared to join the 6th Battalion at Arras. Always concerned about his parents' anxiety, he tried to allay their fears. He wrote:

...you must cheer up and trust in God and our good luck. [...] ... if it pleases God – I am quite ready to go and I could not die a better death and will be proud as you also will be proud for me if necessary to die for England and God's fight against Kulture [sic].[45]

Four days later, he was standing amid light snow in trenches taken over from the French. ETW's anxieties for his son were at least partially assuaged by the knowledge that, as an officer, Bernard enjoyed better living conditions than his men, sleeping in a hut rather than a tent.[46] Nevertheless, by April, Bernard's company was having to cope with the thick mud in the trenches and the discomfort of not being able to change their clothes for six days. On a 'quiet day' when they were not being bombarded by howitzers, they succeeded in killing their first German.[47]

Then, a few days before ETW's golden wedding anniversary, Bernard wrote to his father from a damp dug-out about 15 feet underground. 'The Bosche has not sent any shells over us for the last 24 hours', he wrote. 'They try for our artillery but do not seem to have located them as yet by some hundreds of yards'.[48] Worryingly, the neighbouring village had been totally destroyed, and bombs in the local churchyard had even 'smashed the tomb stones and thrown up the bones and skulls'.[49] As presents and good wishes, including wine sent from Bernard, flooded into *Westal* as part of the celebrations, Bernard was still holed out in the dugout with three comrades. Deep down in cold, wet chalk, they had strengthened the walls with sand bags as occasional shells flew over containing 'yellow poisonous high explosive'.[50] While festivities were muted in the light of ETW's health, the event still drew comment in the *Cheltenham Looker-On*.[51] Toasts to the couple's health were followed by toasts to the rest of the family, including their absentee son on the Western Front. Bernard had promised to be there in spirit, and his mess drank to their health.[52] Despite suffering the discomfort of the dugout, as the coke brazier spewed out pieces of sulphur, Bernard wrote of his deep love for his parents:

> ... you are what you are - the very best and most devoted parents our children could wish to have. You have set us an example – it is very difficult to follow, because it is such a high one. But we are all I know trying to follow in your steps.[53]

Life in Bernard's dug-out proved excellent training in the art of patience, with no-one being able to move an inch without someone else having to shift a little. Having a similarly sustained level of patience was an equally hard lesson for ETW to learn. His pain rarely eased, but amid a sea of despair were occasional islands of calm and hope.

As April showers fell at *Westal*, the trenches again turned to thick mud. Fully aware of the dangers posed by trench foot, ETW was pleased to hear that Bernard was well-equipped with a good pair of boots. By the summer Bernard and his men faced further trials - the scourge of mosquitoes that made their life a misery. ETW sent him various remedies to try, but with mixed success; and the sound of mosquitoes, which Bernard likened to German Fokker aircraft, continued relentlessly.[54]

Still holed down deep in damp chalk and without light (except for a basic paraffin lamp), Bernard wished, despite his own hardship, that he could bear some of his father's pain for him.[55] Then, later, suffering terrible shelling when ten of his men were killed and thirty wounded, Bernard wrote to his father, 'I could feel your prayers all round me and a wonderful feeling of security'.[56]

ETW's letters and cards continued to follow Bernard's movements across France, even though knowledge of specific locations was necessarily strictly embargoed for security reasons. Through Bernard's replies, ETW now learned about the different types of training his company was practising, including bayonet practice, special tactics for fighting in woods, and techniques for advancing through thick undergrowth. What Bernard was recounting were the preparations for the Battle of Delville Wood, a series of engagements that formed part of the Battle of the Somme. His subsequent letters described a series of dramatic incidents: two German prisoners being held by an infantryman with a shattered arm; five British soldiers being blown up by a shell, their remains never recovered; and a man who was so drunk that he had to be left to his fate in a dugout. Bernard did not spare ETW the graphic detail of the horror. Perhaps the worst was how to cope with the stench and the swarms of blue bottles that infested hundreds of dead bodies, which Bernard's men could not bury and upon which they desperately tried to avoid treading. He wrote:

> I do not know if you like to hear these awful details, but it is just as well to let people know, what our men have gone through. So that this shall be the last war in history.[57]

For a time, Bernard seemed to live a charmed life. He was hit on several occasions by pieces of stray shell, but they failed to penetrate his uniform, or else missed a vulnerable part of his body; but then, towards the end of September, worrying news reached *Westal* that Bernard was recovering in hospital after being hit by shrapnel. He had a small, clean wound above his left knee.[58] Yet, despite this, he soon recovered and was even able to make occasional visits home.

In March 1917, thoughts at *Westal* temporarily shifted to Russia and the outbreak of revolution against the government of Tsar Nicholas II. Mary's nephew Jim Whishaw (1853-1935), recently appointed as a supply agent for the Ministry of Munitions, was trying to escape from a detachment of the Red Guards sent to arrest him.[59] He escaped with his life but not his property, and fled Russia for good in October 1917 once Lenin's Bolsheviks overthrew the provisional government.

The following month, when Bernard next visited home, he found his father looking extremely weak and pale. After returning to fight at the Western Front, he encouraged his father likewise to fight on and trust in God's will to give him strength to cope with the pain. Fearing again that his end might be nigh, the day before he received orders to return to France, Bernard paid another tribute to his father:

> You have been the very best of fathers and we have had a truly great example set us by your love, your strenuous activity, your patience and your strength of character. I just want to tell you what you already know that I love, respect and admire you more than anyone I have ever met myself or heard of. Because I know you and your innermost thoughts.[60]

Further letters home described the dangers that Bernard continued to face: in May, he wrote to his father about a British plane that had crashed within 200 yards of him. Bernard helped to recover the pilot, for whose life he was fearful, given that the pilot's bowels were protruding through his torn clothes.[61]

As 1917 drew to a close, Bernard again sensed that his father's remaining days were numbered. 'To my mind there is nothing terrible or terrifying in death,' he wrote on New Year's Eve. 'On the battlefield the dead always seem to me to be so peaceful and almost to be envied – all their work and worry, anxiety and doubt over – their work done and no more pain or tears...' So, too, 'almost with excitement' he anticipated that ETW would meet his end and 'see the great things God has prepared for those who love Him and have served Him',[62] just as ETW had always done.

Nevertheless, ETW's health remained steady, and Bernard, who had applied for a ten-week senior officers' course in Aldershot between January and March, was able to see for himself, during occasional visits to *Westal*, how, at times, his father was relatively strong and free from pain. He was further encouraged by the appointment of a good nurse who assisted his mother and sister Ida with their caring duties.

If ETW's levels of anxiety had subsided during this time, they rose again sharply at the news that Bernard would be immediately returning to the frontline. 'Partings are desperate things,' Bernard wrote to his father at Easter, '...but I know you understand and would have me go out to France and do my share in the great work come what may'.[63] A fortnight later, whilst news from France provided assurance that Bernard was not in imminent danger, ETW suffered another painful attack of fibrositis. Although intense fighting continued in France, Bernard found himself at a loose end: having re-joined his company, which had recently suffered heavy losses, no decision could be taken about how he could be deployed until the reorganisation of the company was complete.

As the fighting raged on, with Bernard beginning to feel increasingly idle, ETW died peacefully in his bed on 19 April, his long fight against pain now at an end. Outside, dragonfly nymphs were beginning to emerge from their larval skins, prior to basking in glorious sunshine. They would soon enjoy the new freedom of flight envisioned in ETW's 'heaven'. Four days later, ETW was laid to rest in an oak coffin beside Nellie and Gwladys in the churchyard of St. Peter's. The simple funeral service was led by his youngest son Jim.[64] Apart from close family, friends and former patients, the mourners included representatives from the organisations with which ETW had been most associated. They included the Delancey Hospital, the Victoria Home, the CNSS, and Friends in Council. The inscription on his gravestone read simply, 'He went about doing good'. Unable to attend the funeral, Bernard imagined his father's 'peaceful dear old face, lying so still and white with his soul and grand old spirit at rest with God'.[65] He felt privileged to have had a father who was 'a splendid example of what a man and a father should be'.[66] Around

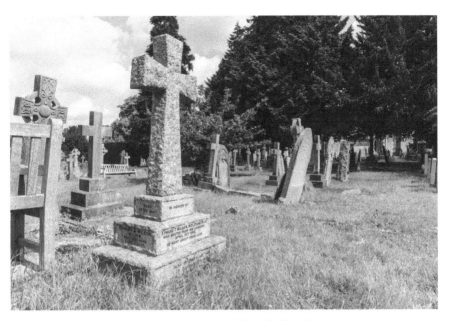

The gravestone at St Peter's Church

six months later, Bernard was also freed of his painful struggle. On 11 November 1918, he wrote to his mother with deep gratitude: 'At last fighting is over … I am safe and sound'.[67]

'Doing Good'

Obituary tributes – Cheltenham's forgotten worthy – Epilogue

'He went about doing good'
~ ETW's epitaph ~

F OLLOWING ETW'S DEATH, SEVERAL tributes appeared in the local press. Unsurprisingly, the two organisations suggested as the most suitable monuments to his memory were the Delancey Hospital, viewed by ETW as 'the most remarkable institution of a philanthropic nature connected with Cheltenham',[1] and the Victoria Home for Nurses: '[They] will always serve to remind the people of Cheltenham of how much they owe to the physician who has now passed away',[2] commented the *Cheltenham Looker-On*. Recognising that he contributed as much to art as to science, it also highlighted the fact that the School of Art '... would have probably collapsed over and over again but for the support he [ETW] gave to it'.[3] As far as his overall contribution was concerned, however, it was perhaps the *Gloucestershire Echo* that summarised this best when it wrote:

> No single man has done more than he – nay, it may be truthfully inserted that none has done so much as he – to stimulate and promote the intellectual life of the town for more than half a century.[4]

Nevertheless, awareness of ETW's considerable achievements soon became forgotten. The reasons why history remembers certain people and overlooks others are complex; and they vary according to the vagaries of changing times and culture. While dying young, or dramatically, has sometimes been a potential tenet of being remembered - in Ted's case as much as General Gordon's - so too, in certain circumstances, has performing notoriously evil acts! Therefore, it is perhaps not surprising that a 'good' doctor initially received only limited recognition. This is especially so when, like his favourite uncle Thomas Bellerby, he performed 'good and great deeds' silently and without ostentation.

His lasting legacy, like ETW himself, is characterised by many subtle and complex dimensions. As a scientist and medical practitioner his ideas were not, in many ways, original for he was generally a seeker of truth,

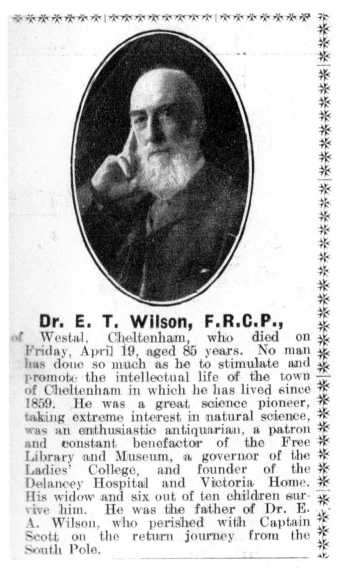

Dr. E. T. Wilson, F.R.C.P.,

of Westal, Cheltenham, who died on Friday, April 19, aged 85 years. No man has done so much as he to stimulate and promote the intellectual life of the town of Cheltenham in which he has lived since 1859. He was a great science pioneer, taking extreme interest in natural science, was an enthusiastic antiquarian, a patron and constant benefactor of the Free Library and Museum, a governor of the Ladies' College, and founder of the Delancey Hospital and Victoria Home. His widow and six out of ten children survive him. He was the father of Dr. E. A. Wilson, who perished with Captain Scott on the return journey from the South Pole.

The obituary from the Cheltenham Chronicle and Gloucestershire Graphic, *4 May 1918.*

not originality. His indefatigable pursuit of accuracy and authenticity manifested itself as much in his scientific work as in other passionate interests, including photomicrography, museum work, and archaeological research. As an expert on what we would now call modern epidemiology, however, there were several examples of adopting innovative approaches - from actively planning the Delancey Hospital from 1871, when the idea of an 'isolation hospital' had only recently started to develop,[5] to conducting pioneering research into the complex interrelationships between different factors governing the health of a town. In the light of the recent coronavirus (COVID-19) pandemic, the relevance of his work on isolation fever hospitals and sanitary statistics deserve to become more widely appreciated.[6] The issues we are grappling with today resonate closely with those occurring 150 years ago, and many of the successful techniques ETW used and promoted then still stand the test of time. His holistic approach for stemming the spread of infectious diseases included campaigns to promote public health and hygiene, including the use of disinfectants; the deployment of front-line nurses in the community to provide early warning indicators; strenuous efforts to supply consistently pure drinking water to the needy; and the prompt isolation of newly identified cases. Regarding the latter, for example, one medical practitioner paid tribute to ETW's 'admirable arrangements at Cheltenham "to isolate *first cases* of the disease, with a view to stopping short an epidemic" ... in the hope that they may be copied by other towns'.[7]

Often working unnoticed in the background, or merely guiding others in certain directions, success for ETW was more about achieving worthy aims than personal satisfaction or glory. While one colleague criticised him for 'often [failing] to carry conviction'[8] in his public speeches, and others that he was 'unobtrusive by nature',[9] there was no doubt that he exercised considerable impact and influence wherever he was present. It was said, '... [he] impressed his personality upon the town's institutions and always for their good'.[10] As President of the local Natural Science Society 'his annual addresses were always marked by keen insight and research'[11] while, as an accomplished naturalist, he contributed invaluable records of the Cheltenham flora and fauna which today provide a benchmark to help us understand the impact of recent environmental changes on local wildlife.

While ETW lived to a grand age, it is remarkable to consider the extraordinary number of distinguished physicians, scientists and other intellectuals that he met throughout his career or counted as his friends - from Francis Frith and Sir William Osler to John Ruskin, to name but a few. The number of new societies he established or contributed to is equally impressive, as too the quantity of papers and articles he produced in his lifetime.[12] His generosity of spirit was also evident in his 'encyclopaedic knowledge'[13] that was always spontaneously given to friends and the townsfolk in general; and, as a collector of books, manuscripts, artwork and other artefacts – from Neolithic flint implements to Woodthorpe's Naga collection – he ensured their long-term preservation for the benefit of the public by transferring them to the most appropriate repositories.

Finally, there is the story of love, devotion and loyalty to his family - well crystallised in the comments made by Bernard from the Western Front. On more than one occasion, he put his family first when making significant decisions, such as whether to accept the BMA Presidency. From a fun-loving Father Christmas, who penned witty verses, to an assiduous biographer, who documented in detail every aspect of his children's lives,[14] ETW provided a strong role model for his children. He passed on to his family a love of learning, nature and art, and a dedication to serve society without ostentation. Ted himself knew how much he owed ETW, not only for the unstinted support he gave to his scientific work[15] but also for the continuous nurturing and development of his interests and skills. He confessed, 'there's no man living I admire so much as him'.[16] He probably reflected on whether he would ever have journeyed to the Antarctic at all were it not for the suggestion of ETW's friend, Dr Sclater, that he should apply for the *Discovery* Expedition's position. Over a century later, however, some recognition was given to ETW when Cheltenham's newly refurbished museum and art gallery was renamed The Wilson following local consultation and public voting for a new name. The Wilson was not just named for Ted but for ETW and other members of the family. Perhaps now, this other Wilson is truly emerging from under the shadows of his more famous son and brother.

~~~

FOLLOWING THE INHERITANCE OF the estate by Mary and the surviving children,[17] the Wilson family remained at *Westal*. Around this time the house became divided into small flats to accommodate Lily's family, and the large garden-level kitchen was transferred into ETW's study.[18] Mary survived ETW by twelve years, and was fondly remembered by members of the family as friendly, kind, thoughtful, intelligent and able to manage 'so many things competently in different spheres'.[19] When she was eventually laid to rest next to ETW and their daughters, it was Jim who, once again, conducted the funeral service at Leckhampton. *Westal* was later sold and then its site re-developed. After ETW's death, Mary ensured that material from his private collections was donated to appropriate institutions. This included, for example, bones that ETW had acquired from the Long Barrow at West Tump, in Brimpsfield, and artefacts from Cleeve Hill Camp, all of which Mary subsequently donated to the town museum. Following the First World War, Bernard returned to Yorkshire to work as a land agent. He received a Distinguished Service Order (D.S.O.) in the 1919 King's birthday honours list and, for a while, given that he was 'always full of fun of one kind or another',[20] carried on ETW's tradition of playing Father Christmas in full dress at *Westal*. For Jim, it was a different story. Scarred by his experience as a chaplain serving with soldiers from South Staffordshire on the Western Front, but also transformed after seeing a vision of Christ calling him to work with the poor, he became involved in the Catholic Crusade. This led him to seek radical political reform to combat poverty and deprivation in the Potteries and elsewhere. Later, as chaplain to The Guild of Health, he founded Edward Wilson House in Queen Anne Street, London as a memorial to Ted, where he promoted reconciliation and healing. The last member of the Wilson family to live in Cheltenham was Ida, who died in 1963. For much of her life, she cared for her sister Elsie who suffered from poor health, including mental difficulties. The Wilson family nevertheless maintains its links with the town, principally through the family archive deposited with the museum, an institution which Edward Thomas Wilson was proud to open over 110 years ago.

Notes

Notes to Chapter 1

1   Wesley Street in the Princes Park, Toxteth area of Liverpool was laid out in 1826, so the Wilsons' home was then very new. The area has since been completely redeveloped, the site being now occupied by Corinto Street.

2   E.T. Wilson, *My Life. Volume I: 1832-1888. Volume II: 1889-1916.* Illustrated, hand-written. Two black leather volumes with gold lettering, Cheltenham Borough Council and the Cheltenham Trust/The Wilson Family Collection (Ref. 1995.550.35 A & B), p.1. Subsequent references to these volumes are indicated by *ML*.

3   ETW's godfathers were the partners in the Anglo-American banking houses, William Brown, later Sir William Brown (1784-1864) and Joseph Shipley (1795-1867), the latter subsequently settling in the USA.

4   Hean Castle, or *Hen Gastell* (Welsh for 'old castle') as it was originally known, was first mentioned in 1295. In 1358, it came under the ownership of Laurence de Hastings, Earl of Pembroke and was called Hengastel. In 1800, when the Stokes acquired the estate, it consisted of a mansion, the lordship of St Issels and Treberth, a castle mill and twenty-one farms. For further information see Francis Jones, *Historic Houses of Pembrokeshire and their families*, (Brawdy Books, 1996).

5   Dr E.T. Wilson, 'The Family Faculties Book' [A record of family members and characteristics drafted by Dr E.T. Wilson of Cheltenham (1832-1918) as part of early research into genetic inheritance by Francis Galton FRS], Cheltenham Borough Council and the Cheltenham Trust/The Wilson Family Collection (Ref. 1995.550.61), p.5.

6   *ML*, pp.8-9.

7   ETW was so fond of the Giant's Causeway stones that he later transferred them to his garden in Cheltenham.

8   *ML*, pp.18-19.

9   Ibid., p.17.

10   Ibid., p.29.

11   Ibid., p.25.

12   Ibid., p.34.

13   Ibid., p.27.

14   Ibid., p.32.

15   William Keatley Stride, *Exeter College* (F.E. Robinson and Co., 1900), p.177.

16   *ML*, p.36.

17   Ibid., p.41.

18   Ibid.

19   Ibid., p.42.

20 Ibid., p.38.
21 Ibid., pp.43-44.
22 Ibid., p.44.
23 *Pembrokeshire Herald and General Advertiser*, 30 June 1854, p.2, col. 6.
24 When the house was built at the beginning of the nineteenth century new silver flatware would have been ordered to grace the tables of the house. One spoon hallmarked 1804 survives today. It was made by a journeyman in the London workshops of William Eley and William Fearn who were regarded as the finest silversmiths of their day. Information supplied by Gary Davies, a local historian with a special interest in Hean Castle.
25 *ML*, p.47.
26 The house was called Clifton House at the time of ETW's visit, later Edginswell, now Windsor House.
27 *ML*, p.50.
28 Ibid., p.51.
29 Ibid.
30 Ibid., p.53.
31 Ibid., p.61.
32 Ibid., p.62.
33 William Ogle (1827-1912) was one of ETW's Oxford friends and a fellow student at St George's. Later, he taught physiology at St George's, and then became Superintendent of Statistics at the Registrar-General.
34 *ML*, p.72.
35 Ibid.
36 Ibid., p.73.
37 Ibid., p.75.
38 Ibid., p.74. Caesar Hawkins (1798-1884) and Sir Benjamin Collins Brodie (1783-1862) were both noted for their conservative approach. Hawkins encouraged his students to always try to save a limb, rather than remove it unnecessarily, and Brodie's pioneering research into bone and joint disease resulted led to a reduced number of amputations being carried out by surgeons.
39 Ibid., p.75.
40 Ibid., p.78.
41 Rowland Fothergill (1794-1871) had the reputation of being an able iron-master. The Taff Vale iron-works, which was one of several that he owned in the area, was located in the parish of Llantwit Fardre, near Pontypridd.

Notes to Chapter 2
1 The authors of these testimonials included Physicians at St. George's Hospital, King's College Hospital, and Oxford's Radcliffe Infirmary as well as Dr Henry Acland, Regius Professor of Medicine, Oxford, and Dr Philip Sclater, Secretary of the Zoological Society.
2 See the obituary of John Abercrombie, M.D. in the *Medico-Chirurgical Transactions* (vol. 76, 1893), p.28.

3   See *Transactions of Cheltenham College Boat Club*, 1860, Cheltenham College Archives (Ref. C315/CS).

4   *ML*, p.93.

5   Ibid., p.92. The Association, whose objective was achieved within five years, was founded on 7 November 1861, primarily with a focus on botanical work. However, since similar work was needed for the county the association was subsequently merged into a new society called the Cheltenham and Gloucestershire Naturalists' Association. For more information see Gloucestershire Archives (see Ref. D11752).

6   Dr. E.T. Wilson, 'Inaugural Address', *Proceedings of Cheltenham Natural Science Society*, 1892-93, p.5.

7   In 1906, he read a paper on Diatomaceae for the Cheltenham Natural Science Society. See Dr.E.T.Wilson, 'The Diatomaceae', *Cheltenham Examiner*, 31 October 1906, p.2, cols.6-7.

8   For a detailed description of the expedition see chapter 2 of Charles M. Watson's biography, *The Life of Major-General Sir Charles William Wilson* (John Murray, 1909).

9   The medical library was first established at the hospital and subsequently transferred to the Royal Crescent library, Thomas's the Chemist and, lastly, the town library.

10 Major General Sir Frederick Carrington acquired fame as the military leader who helped to crush the 1896 Matabele rebellion. He was also a friend of Cecil Rhodes.

11 *ML*, p.96.

12 Ibid., p.100.

13 'Hean Castle Estate', *Welshman*, 11 September 1863, p.5, col.5.

14 Countess Stenbock was the daughter of Johan Frerichs, a Manchester cotton industrialist who had originally emigrated from Bremen. The family built Thirlestaine Hall in 1855-7 in Bath Road, Cheltenham where her son, the poet and writer of fantastic fiction Count Eric Stanislaus Stenbock (1860-95), was born.

15 Today, this is located on Montpellier Spa Road.

16 See [Edward T. Wilson], 'Death certificates and the registration of disease', in *British and Foreign Medico-Chirurgical Review* vol. 44 (July-October 1869), pp. 294-315.

17 Ibid., p.297.

18 See Edward Wilson, 'Sanitary statistics of Cheltenham' in *Report of the Thirty-Fourth Meeting of the British Association for the Advancement of Science held at Bath in September 1864* (John Murray, 1865), pp. 180-183.

19 'The fallacies and shortcomings of our sanitary statistics', in *Social Science Review* vol. 4 (July to December 1865), p 236.

20 [Edward T. Wilson], 'Death certificates and the registration of disease', p.306.

21 Ibid., p.306.

22 Ibid., p.307.

Notes to Chapter 3

1   *ML*, p.106.

2   It is the sixth oldest, excluding London (founded in 1853), which became The Royal Photographic Society. In 1936 it renamed itself Cheltenham Camera Club and currently has around 130 members.

3   Jean-Claude Lemagny and André Rouillé, *A history of photography: social and cultural perspectives* (Cambridge University Press, 1986), p.30.

4   [Edward Thomas Wilson], 'Photomicrography', *British and Foreign Medico-Chirurgical Review* vol.34 (July-October 1864), p.2.

5   Ibid.

6   The Cheltenham studio had another important connection. Its ownership was later transferred to Richard Beard, the son of the sole patentee of the daguerreotype process in England and Wales, also called Richard, who had set up Europe's first public photographic studio at the Royal Polytechnic Institution in Regent Street, London on 23 March 1841.

7   The event was reported with some solemnity by the local press: 'On Monday the first day of the institute being opened, the weather was lovely and a great many of our leading gentry honoured Mr. Palmer by sitting to his invisible artiste, and in all cases the sitters were presented with undeniable references to their own personal identity. Nothing can exceed the fidelity with which the minutiae of feature, dress and posture are represented by this talismanic process. We can conceive nothing more pleasurable than the feelings of a distant relative or friend on receiving one of these exquisite mementoes from those who are dear to us.' *Cheltenham Examiner*, 15 September 1841, p.3 col.5.

8   'Electro-Enamelled Daguerreotypes', *Cheltenham Journal and Gloucestershire Fashionable Weekly Gazette*, 20 November 1852, p.3, col.3.

9   Lowe claimed, for example, that the chemicals he used and the way in which he applied them improved the brilliancy of tone and colour of the daguerreotype; also, the thickness of the silver he used helped to produce 'an image rich, clear, brilliant, and distinctly developed in every part of the folds and drapery'; and its gilding with chloride of gold helped to protect it from sun-light. See 'Electro Enamelled Daguerreotype by a new process', *Cheltenham Examiner*, 14 April 1852, p.8, col.3.

10 While other sources claim that Lowe ran into financial difficulty the *Cheltenham Journal* reported, 'It is understood that the defaulter had a most successful business, and that his pecuniary circumstances were in the most satisfactory condition, and the proceeding is rendered, therefore, the more inexplicable.' See *Cheltenham Journal and Gloucestershire Fashionable Weekly Gazette*, 1 November 1856, p.2, col.3.

11 Simon Fletcher, 'Cheltenham's first photographers 1841-1856', *Cheltenham Local History Society Journal* vol. 3 (1985), p.24.

12 Sue Rowbotham and Jill Waller, *Cheltenham: a history* (Phillimore, 2004), p.69.

13 Simon Fletcher, p.24.

14 'Cheltenham Amateur Photographic Society. A Successful Revival', *Gloucestershire Echo*, 29 January 1909, p.3, col. 2.

15 Bill Jay, *Victorian cameraman; Francis Frith's views of rural England, 1850-1898* (David & Charles, 1973), p.26.

16 *ML*, p.28.

17 Ibid., p.52.

18 Lemagny and Rouillé, *A history of photography*, p.71.

19 R. Derek Wood, 'J.B. Reade, F.R.S., and the early history of photography. Part 1. A re-assessment on the discovery of contemporary evidence', *Annals of Science*, vol. 27, no. 1 (March 1971), p. 29.

20 Edward T. Wilson, 'How to photograph microscopic objects', *Popular Science Review*, vol. 6 1867, p. 54.

21 Ibid., p. 55.

22 Apart from being a physician Dr Maddox was a leading expert in photomicrography. He was also famous for paving the way for the replacement of the wet collodion plates with the dry plate process using gelatine.

23 Edward T. Wilson, 'How to photograph microscopic objects', p. 55.

24 Lionel Smith Beale, *How to work with the microscope*, (Harrison 1868), 4th ed., pp. 247-249.

25 Ibid., pp. 248-9.

26 Ibid., p.249.

27 For further information on photozincography see John Hannavy (ed.), *Encyclopedia of nineteenth-century photography*, (Taylor & Francis, 2008), p.1119.

28 [Edward Thomas Wilson], Photomicrography, *British and Foreign Medico-Chirurgical Review* vol.34 (July-October 1864), p.25.

Notes to Chapter 4

1 For a detailed account see David O'Connor and Ian Harvey, *Troubled Waters: the great Cheltenham water controversy* (David O'Connor, 2007).

2 Ibid., p.2.

3 Sue Rowbotham and Jill Waller, *Cheltenham: a history* (Phillimore, 2004), p.93.

4 'The rival water schemes', *Cheltenham Looker-On* 25 February 1865, p.120.

5 The strapline of the *Cheltenham Examiner* was 'Intelligence, integrity and independence'.

6 Edward T. Wilson, 'Consideration of the introduction of Severn water for the supply of the town', *Cheltenham Examiner*, 27 February 1865.

7 *ML*, p.109.

8 The lecture was given on 26 April 1865.

9 'Water in its relation to health', *Cheltenham Examiner*, 26 April 1865, p.6, cols.1-3.

10 Ibid.

11 Ibid.

12 See 'Cheltenham water supply. Enquiry before the Lords', *Cheltenham*

Examiner 14 June 1865, p.8, cols.3-4. Note: ETW is wrongly referred to as 'Dr. Williams'.

Notes to Chapter 5

1   The Assembly Rooms were located on the corner of Rodney Road, its site now occupied by Lloyd's Bank.
2   See *Cheltenham Looker-On*, 28 January 1865, p.9, col.2.
3   See account of the Bachelors' Ball on 14 February 1843 referred to in Daniel L. Lipson, *About and around Cheltenham*, 10th ed. (Ed. J. Burrow & Co. Ltd, c.1949), p.24.
4   Quoted descriptions of the Bachelors' Ball are taken from *Cheltenham Examiner*, 1 March 1865, p.8, cols.1-3 and *Cheltenham Looker-On*, 4 March 1865, pp.135-8.
5   *ML*, p.112.
6   Ibid.
7   Ibid., p.114.
8   Ibid., p.116.
9   Ibid.
10 John Goding, *History of Cheltenham* (Longman, 1853), p.213.
11 Located in College Lawn, Linden House (now known as Queen's House) is used as a girls' day house at Cheltenham College.
12 'Mother of famous explorer: Mrs. Wilson's death in Cheltenham', *Cheltenham Chronicle*, 25 October 1930, p.4, col.4.
13 It is interesting to note that a Ladies' Friends in Council was established on 11 April 1872, and Mary Agnes Wilson was appointed as its honorary secretary. See *ML*, p.139.
14 When Friends in Council was founded Barnard lived in Cambridge House, in St George's Road. Later he moved to Bartlow on Leckhampton Hill. For a summary of his life, see David O'Connor, 'Major Robert Cary Barnard, 1827-1906', *Leckhampton Local History Society Research Bulletin*, No.4 (Summer 2010), pp.7-12.
15 Sir Arthur Helps, *Friends in Council, a Series of Readings and Discourse thereon* (1847-1859), 2 vols.
16 *Friends in Council, list of members and papers read at their meetings in fifty years, 1862-1912*, [1912], p.3.
17 Henry James was also the inventor of the first portable folding chair. See *English Patents of Inventions, Specifications A.D.1867, 1st January No.6*, pp.1-6.
18 From 1869 to 1911, ETW presented the following thirty-four papers at Friends in Council meetings: 'Charles Waterton' (1869); 'Life of Edward Forbes, the Naturalist' (1870); 'The Morality of Field Sports' (1871); 'Phrenology and Physiognomy' (1872); 'The Expression of the Emotions' (1873); 'The Heredity of Mental Qualities' (1874); 'Cave Hunting' (1875); 'Vivisection' (1876); 'Marquis of Worcester and Century of Inventions' (1877); 'Colour in Plants and Animals' (1879); 'Sir Thomas Browne's Pseudodoxia Epidemica' (1881); 'Aristotle's Parts of Animals' (1883); 'Human Faculty (Galton)' (1884); 'Duality

of Mind' (1885); 'Poems of O. W. Holmes' (1886); 'Popular Government (India)' (1887); 'Hypnotism' (1889); 'Motley's Correspondence' (1890); 'Hereditary Aptitudes' (1891); 'The Naturalist in La Plata (Hudson)' (1892); 'A Forecast of National Life and Character' (1893); 'Merrie England' (1895); 'Jenner and his work' (1896); 'William Harvey' (1898); 'Temperaments up to date' (1899); 'Bloch's Modern Weapons and Modern War' (1900); 'Some usages of war, with special reference to international law' (1901);) 'The Authorship of Shakespeare' (1902; 'Antarctic Experiences of the Discovery' (1904); 'The Mind's Eye' (1905); 'Man and Evolution' (1907); 'Finger Prints' (1908); 'The Power of Visualisation' (1909); 'A neglected inheritance of blood' (1911). Information taken from *Friends in Council, list of members and papers read at their meetings in fifty years, 1862-1912*, [1912]. A more recent index compiled by the Friends in Council archivist lists 38 papers in total, including an early paper on the Duke of Argyll's 'Reign of Law' and later papers on 'Flints and men of the Cotswolds' and 'A journey in Antarctic night'.

19 *ML*, p.134.
20 *ML*, pp.134-5.
21 After leaving Cheltenham to become Headmaster of Bradfield College and then Rugby School, he dedicated his book on the voyage of Jason to 'his "Friends in Council" at Cheltenham, in memory of many delightful and profitable hours spent in their society ...'. See Henry Hayman, *A Fragment of the Iason Legend: The Earlier Portions Republished from the 'Contemporary Review'*, (James Parker and Company, 1871).
22 Quoted in Josephine Butler, *Recollections of George Butler*, (J.W. Arrowsmith, 1892), p. 137.
23 Ibid.

Notes to Chapter 6

1 The rest of ETW's witty poem reads: 'She is neat and tidy and trim as can be / A soothing sight for the sick to see / With a sweet low voice and a gentle touch / She comforts the patient just as much / Possibly more than the Doctor's potions / Or the diligent rubbing of all his lotions / So I've bought her a book which may help to cheer / Long hours of watch in the coming year'. This poem was penned during December 1886 when a nurse called Mary Jones came to stay at *Westal*. It accompanied ETW's Christmas present of a book to her. See *ML*, p.193.
2 'An evening with Charles Dickens', *Cheltenham Chronicle*, 26 January 1869, p.5, col.3.
3 For a description of Sarah Gamp see Charles Dickens, *The Life and Adventures of Martin Chuzzlewit*, (Chapman and Hall, 1874 [first published 1842-44], p.379.
4 *ML*, p.121.
5 'Cheltenham Nursing Institution', *Cheltenham Examiner*, 29 March 1871, p.4 col.6.
6 'County Nursing Association', *Cheltenham Examiner*, 1 July 1909, p.7, col.3-5.

7   Ibid.
8   Ibid.
9   As an example, ETW said, 'If they had on the Committee a masterful mind
    that dictated too much, that left the doctor out of the question, and even
    went so far as to say the nurse was more important than the doctor; or if
    they had a doctor who was touchy and resented what the nurse did and was
    inclined to think the nurse was doing work which he alone ought to do; or if
    they had a nurse who of set purpose took some of the doctor's work into her
    own hands - out of any one of these circumstances, difficulties might arise
    which it would need a lot of tact to compose'. Ibid.
10 *ML*, p.121.
11 'An unfounded rumour', *Cheltenham Examiner*, 5 August 1868, p.4, col.5.
12 Ibid.
13 The inn, first recorded in 1834, was located at 140 Bath Road.
14 'Death of a flyman: extraordinary enquiry', *Cheltenham Examiner*, 12 August
    1868, p.2, cols.1-4.
15 *ML*, pp.125-6.
16 *Cheltenham Times and Record*, 8 August 1868.
17 *ML*, p.126.
18 Edward T. Wilson, 'The deficiency of the water supply of the town', *Cheltenham
    Examiner*, 10 March 1869, p.8 col.4. Also published in *Cheltenham Chronicle*,
    16 March 1869, p.5, col. 4.
19 Ibid.
20 Ibid.
21 Ibid.
22 'The Palestine Exploration Fund', *Cheltenham Examiner*, 17 November 1869,
    p.8, cols.1-2.
23 Edward T. Wilson, 'Notes on the Subcutaneous Injection of Morphia', *St.
    George's Hospital Report*, 4 (1869), p.30. It is also worth noting that ETW's
    assertion was well-founded. See, for example, Terry Parssinen's comment:
    'In the same year [that ETW published his review into the possible uses of
    injected morphia], Dr. Arthur Evershed chided his "professional brethren"
    whose misplaced caution about injected morphia kept them from using this
    "means of relief so satisfactory to their patients and to themselves"'. See
    Terry M. Parssinen, *Secret Passions, Secret Remedies: Narcotic Drugs in British
    Society, 1820-1930*, (Manchester University Press, 1983), p.80.

Notes to Chapter 7
1   E.T.Wilson, 'The plague of 1871 in Buenos Ayres', *Food Journal*, vol.3 (1
    February 1872), p.21.
2   After returning home, Harry became Secretary to the Gardner's Trust for
    the Blind and founded a magazine for the blind, the first of its kind in the
    English-speaking world, which he edited for twenty-two years.
3   W. H. Illingworth, *History of the Education of the Blind*, London: Sampson Low,
    Marston & Company, Ltd., 1910, p. 154.

4   E.T.Wilson, 'The plague of 1871 in Buenos Ayres', p.19.
5   Ibid., p.20.
6   Ibid., p.22.
7   For a report of the meeting see 'A fever hospital for Cheltenham', *Cheltenham Examiner* 19 April 1871, p.8, cols. 2-4.
8   An original suggestion to build the hospital on a vacant site in Swindon Road, adjacent to the Poor Law Infirmary, led to controversy 'as its proximity would be bound to taint it with the Poor Law'. See Heather Atkinson, *Cheltenham: a case study in hospital provision 1918-1948*. A thesis submitted to the University of Gloucestershire in accordance with the requirements for the degree of Masters of Arts in the Faculty of Humanities. 2004, p.65.
9   E.T.Wilson, *Disinfectants and how to use them*, (H.K. Lewis: [1871]).
10   See, for example, the following reviews reproduced in the advert in Louis C. Parkes, *Infectious diseases, notification and prevention* (Royal College of Physicians of Edinburgh: 1894), p.207: '"The information given is exact and full, a remarkable amount of knowledge being compressed within a little room." - *British Medical Journal*. "This is an excellent little card-booklet of four pages, containing:- (1) a good list of disinfectants and antiseptics; (2) information as to their special use, and (3) general directions, with regard to disinfection after and during a case of infectious disease. Everyone who is brought in contact with infectious disease in any form should possess this helpful little card. It will be found to be of great practical use, and the price is so small that local boards should be able to distribute it widely." - *Sanitary Record*. "The card cannot but prove useful and every educated householder should have a copy within easy reach in his house." *Medical Press*. "The information is up to date and concisely conveyed." - *Health*. "In households where infectious disease has broken out these cards should be useful and valuable." - *Chemist and Druggist*.'
11   *ML*, p.139.
12   Ibid., p.140.
13   Ibid.
14   Edward T. Wilson, 'Sanitary statistics of Cheltenham for the years 1865-71 inclusive', in *British Medical Journal* 7 September 1872, p.268.

Notes to Chapter 8
1   Recording of an interview between Dr David Wilson and Peter Rendall, together with his sister Betty, at Chippings, 155 The Hill, Burford on 21 September 1996. Cheltenham Borough Council and the Cheltenham Trust/ The Wilson Family Collection.
2   Ibid.
3   Bernhard Fock, the Dutch Inspector of the Russian Imperial Gardens, became William Whishaw's father-in-law after his marriage to Constancia Fock in 1777. Berhard also oversaw the Imperial greenhouses which produced the first peach ever grown in Russia. See Marie-Louise Karttunen, 'Making a communal world: English Merchants in Imperial St. Petersburg', (Faculty of

Social Sciences, University of Helsinki: 2005), p.11. Note: it was erroneously reported in the *Cheltenham Chronicle* obituary of Mary (see 'Mother of famous explorer: Mrs. Wilson's death in Cheltenham', *Cheltenham Chronicle*, 25 October 1930, p.4, col.4) that it was Mary's grandfather, rather than Bernhard Fock, who laid out the Peterhof Gardens for the Russian Czar.

4   Bernhard and some other Whishaw relatives are buried at St Peter's Church, Leckhampton. See Eric Miller, 'Eminent Cheltonians commemorated at Leckhampton', *Cheltenham Local History Society Journal* vol. 23 (2007) pp. 24-5.

5   James Whishaw, *A History of the Whishaw Family*, (Methuen: 1935), p.140.

6   Ibid., p.171.

7   *ML*, p.142.

8   Writing at the end of the nineteenth century Fred Whishaw provided the following description: 'On the left bank of the river [Ochta at Mourino] a colony of English residents have for about a century been established. They have built themselves beautiful houses, and laid out gardens which any English gardener might be proud to claim as the product of his skill. They have English boats on the river, English dogs bark at you as you approach the extensive grounds, English voices greet you everywhere, and English children may be seen playing at English games: it is a bit of England. The colony establishes itself here every summer, coming down from St. Petersburg about May, and returning to town about the end of August. Speaking as one who knows it well, I may say that Mourino is one of the most delightful places in the world'. See Frederick Whishaw, *Out of Doors in Tsarland* (Longmans, Green, and Co., 1893), p.40.

9   James Whishaw, p.171.

10 This was the description of him by his brother Bernard. See James Whishaw, p.170.

11 Eric Miller, 'Dr Wilson and his friends', *Cheltenham Local History Society Journal* vol. 35 (2019), p.15.

12 James Whishaw, pp.140-1.

13 *ML*, p.143.

14 It is likely that the hospital in question was the Prince Oldenburg Children's Hospital, built during 1867-69, which ETW refers to in his paper 'Isolation as a means of arresting epidemic disease', read before the Health Section of the Social Science Association in 1878.

15 Edward T. Wilson, 'Questions connected with vaccination', *St George's Hospital Reports* vol. 7 (1872-4), p.1.

16 Ibid., p.2.

17 J.A. Dudgeon, 'Development of smallpox vaccine in England in the eighteenth and nineteenth centuries', *British Medical Journal* (25 May 1963), p.1369.

18 Edward T. Wilson, 'Animal vaccination', *British Medical Journal*, Vol. 1, No. 842 (17 February 1877), p. 216.

19 A recent history of smallpox notes that 'Arm-to-arm vaccination had begun in 1801, at the St. Petersburg Foundling Hospital after the empress obtained

lymph from Jenner and was continued until 1867, when vaccine from cows was utilized. During the years 1826-1846, there were 17 epidemics of smallpox: out of approximately 15,000 foundlings vaccinated, only 34 developed smallpox, with only one fatality.' See S. L. Kotar and J. E. Gessler, *Smallpox: A History*, (McFarland & Co., 2012), p.70.

20 Edward T. Wilson, 'Questions connected with vaccination', p.14.

21 Ibid., p.12.

22 Ibid., p.9.

23 J.A. Dudgeon, p.1367.

24 In February 1872, Mary received a letter from her brother Bernard (incidentally, a friend of Tsar Nicholas II) and giving her the following message: 'Tell Jim that Willie shot a fine wolf last Sunday at Ostromancha by means of driving through the woods and twisting a little dog's tail. Jim will be pleased to hear it because it is such an unusual chance: people go 50 times upon this intellectual sort of sport, and don't get a chance, and here is this boy goes once and gets a pop at them immediately'. See James Whishaw, *A History of the Whishaw Family*, (Methuen, 1935), p.167.

25 *ML*, p.145.

Notes to Chapter 9

1   'The "Bore" in the Severn', *Globe*, 18 April 1874, p.3, col.2.

2   The physician in question was Dr. Disney L. Thorp who worked at Cheltenham General Hospital.

3   *ML*, p.148.

4   As a tribute to the Revd James Henry Leigh Gabell's generous support for the Delancey Fever Hospital, a portrait of him painted by Edwin Williams (1822–1881) was presented to the hospital in 1877. It showed him holding the ground plan of the hospital in his hands against the background of a fresco painting of the Good Samaritan. See 'A generous gift', *Cheltenham Examiner*, 17 October 1877, p.8, col.5. By 1881, Gabell had donated nearly £10,000 to the hospital. See 'The princely munificence of the Rev. J. H. Gabell', *Cheltenham Looker-On*, 15 October 1881, p.7, cols.1-2. The fact that his father had been a doctor (at Cowes, the Isle of Wight) might explain his interest in health.

5   *ML*, p.148.

6   Ibid.

7   Ibid, p.149.

8   The Delancey Fever Hospital, *Cheltenham Examiner*, 3 February 1875, p.4 col.6.

9   'The Delancey Hospital', *Cheltenham Examiner*, 9 March 1898, p.2, cols.5-7.

10 Ibid.

11 'The treatment of Scarlatina patients', *Cheltenham Examiner*, 18 November 1874, p.8, col.6.

12 Ibid.

13 It is thought that the museum was established largely at the instigation of

Charles Pierson, a Director of the College from 1856-62 and, later, a Member of the College Council from 1862-83. He donated his large geological collection to form the basis of the museum. Upon his resignation in 1883, for failing health, it was decided that the museum should be called the Pierson Museum, and that he should be the honorary curator. (Information provided by Cheltenham College Archives).

14 In a letter dated 6 Oct 1883 ETW wrote: 'The ovaries are well shown and an egg fully formed in situ. The jar is only half filled with fluid but all seems well prepared' (see Dr E.T. Wilson, Letter [to Hunterian Museum], 6 October 1883, Royal College of Surgeons (RCS archive ref. RCS-MUS/5/2/4). Unfortunately, the specimen (listed under the collection reference OC3382A) is no longer present in the RCS collection. The College was bombed in May 1941, and up to three-quarters of the collections were destroyed. It appears that it may have perished then.

15 *ML*, p.154.

16 See 'Death of Mr. Perton, of Prestbury', *Cheltenham Examiner*, 9 November 1881, p.8 col.1, and 'The late Mr. George Perton', *Cheltenham Examiner*, 16 November 1881, p.8, col. 1.

17 *ML*, p.171.

18 Ibid., p.173.

19 Ibid., p.165.

20 Queen Victoria's Journals, Reference RA VIC/MAIN/QVJ (W) Journal Entry: Friday 14th November 1879. http://www.queenvictoriasjournals.org/home.do. Retrieved 7 March 2020.

21 Their friendship was probably strengthened when, for a time, Rumsey lived at The Priory where ETW held his practice.

22 *ML*, p.152.

23 *ML*, p.156.

24 'The Delancey Fever Hospital', *Cheltenham Examiner*, 11 April 1877, p.4, cols.5-6.

25 Edward T. Wilson, 'Isolation as a means of arresting epidemic disease', *Practitioner* (February 1879), p.142.

26 'The Delancey Hospital', *Cheltenham Examiner*, 9 March 1898, p.2, cols.5-7.

27 Ibid.

Notes to Chapter 10

1 'Practical hints on health', *Cheltenham Examiner*, 18 October 1876, p.2, cols.4-6.

2 Born in Cheltenham in 1837, James Winterbotham became a solicitor, serving in the family firm. From 1881 he became an Alderman and also served as a J.P. ETW and Winterbotham became friends through their membership of Friends in Council. They also shared several interests, including fine art and philanthropic work.

3 'The battle of the waters - a legend', *Cheltenham Examiner*, 10 April 1878 p.8, col.3.

4   'The Cheltenham water question', *Cheltenham Examiner*, 13 March 1878, p.8, cols.1-3.

5   'The organisation of charity', *Cheltenham Examiner*, 18 June 1879, p. 8, col.4.

6   *ML*, p.166.

7   'Nurses for the poor', *Cheltenham Examiner*, 12 May 1880, p.8, col.6.

8   Ibid.

9   'Charity Organization Society', *Cheltenham Chronicle*, 9 November 1880, p.5, cols.1-3.

10   *ML*, p.170.

11   Ibid., pp.169-170.

12   In 1888, the farm buildings comprised: 'Loose Box and Trap House, with Loft over, covered in Yard, Calf House, Two Cow Sheds, capable of accommodating 8 Cows, with Meal House adjoining; also Pig-stye with Yard'.See 'Sales particulars for Sunnymeade', Engall and Sanders. Cheltenham, 15 March 1888 (Gloucestershire Archives Ref. D22992633 7/146/1.

13   Interestingly, ETW's survey identified that some health authorities even paid the wages of the infected patients who were admitted to their hospitals, similar in practice to the recent Covid furlough scheme.

14   Edward T. Wilson, 'Isolation as a means of arresting epidemic disease', *Practitioner* (February 1879), p.142.

15   Here, he gave daily consultations (Monday to Saturday from 0900 to 1100, 1400-1500 and 1800 to 2000; Sundays 0900-1000, 1700-1800). If requested, he also made house visits at all hours.

16   The Baron stated that his initial stance was designed not to 'alienate all the moderate pro-vaccinators, [and] numbers of good Liberals'. (see 'Anti-vaccination', *Cheltenham Mercury*, 21 February 1880, p.2, col.7).

17   See 'The Baron de Ferrieres and the Anti-vaccinators', *Cheltenham Mercury*, 20 March 1880, p.3, col.4.

18   'Dr Jenner in Cheltenham', *Cheltenham Examiner*, 7 January 1880, p. 6, col.2.

19   When Jenner resided at No. 8. St.George's Place, Cheltenham, he wrote on 6 November 1810, 'My two eldest children were inoculated for the smallpox before I began to inoculate for the cowpox. My youngest child was born about the time my experiments commenced, and was among the first I ever vaccinated. By referring to the first work I published on the subject in the Spring of the year 1798, page 40, you will find his name Robt. F. Jenner, and you will observe it noticed that on his arm the vaccine lymph did not prove infectious. It advanced two or three days and then died away. In a short time after I was necessitated to go with my family to Cheltenham for a few months, where I did not think it prudent to resume my operations, from a supposition that the people assembled at a watering place might conceive the disease (then so little known) to be contagious, and it might excite a clamour. However, during my stay here, this boy was accidentally exposed to the smallpox, and in such a way as to leave no doubt on my mind of his being infected. Having at this time no vaccine matter in my possession, there was no alternative but his immediate inoculation, which was done by Mr.

Cother, a surgeon of this place, who is since dead, but this history is well known to many who are living. You now see on what a baseless foundation the insinuations which have been published respecting those facts rest'. See 'Dr Jenner in Cheltenham', *Cheltenham Examiner*, 7 January 1880, p.6, col.2.

20 For a summary of the event see 'Conversazione', *Cheltenham Examiner*, 22 June 1881, p.3, cols.4-6.

21 The condition is known as Brown-Séquard syndrome.

22 See 'On men of science, their nature and their nurture'. *Proceedings of the Royal Institution of Great Britain*. Vol. 7 (1874), pp. 227–36.

23 For example, ETW presented the following papers on the subject: 'Heredity of mental qualities' (1874) to Friends in Council; 'Heredity in man controllable by Man' (1889) to the Cheltenham Debating Society; 'Hereditary aptitudes' (1891) to the Cheltenham Natural Science Society; and 'Our inheritance' (1910) to the Cheltenham Natural Science Society.

24 Dr E.T.Wilson, 'Record of Family Faculties' [A record of family members and characteristics drafted by Dr E.T.Wilson of Cheltenham (1832-1918) as part of early research into genetic inheritance by Francis Galton FRS], Cheltenham Borough Council and the Cheltenham Trust/The Wilson Family Collection (Ref. 1995.550.61).

Notes to Chapter 11

1 *ML*, p.185.

2 'Latest telegrams from Egypt. The advance across the desert', *Cheltenham Looker-On*, 3 January 1885, p.12, cols.1-2.

3 The telegram is quoted in 'War in Egypt – Fall of Khartoum', *Cheltenham Looker-On*, 7 February 1885, p.7, cols 1-2.

4 The first news of Gordon's death arrived via a telegram in London on 5 February, but his death was not confirmed until days later.

5 Mike Snook, *Wolseley, Wilson and the failure of the Khartoum Campaign: An Exercise in Scapegoating and Abrogation of Command Responsibility?*, Cranfield University, 2004 PhD Thesis, p.67. In his thesis Snook concludes 'that the failure occurred at the operational level of war, not the tactical; and that accordingly culpability should properly be attributed to Wolseley' (see p.3).

6 The note reads: 'From General Lord Wolseley to the Secretary of State for War. CAIRO, April 13th, 1885. My LORD, I have the honour to forward a letter from Colonel Sir C. Wilson, R.E., giving the reasons for the delay in the departure of the steamers from Gubat. I do not propose to add any remarks of my own to this letter. The reasons given by Sir Charles Wilson must speak for themselves. I have, etc., WOLSELEY, General'. Quoted in C.M. Watson, *The Life of Major-General Sir Charles Wilson*, John Murray, 1909, p.338.

7 See Mike Snook, p.116.

8 The letter was also reproduced in the *Gloucestershire Echo*. See 'Notes and Comments', *Gloucestershire Echo*, 8 May 1885, p.2, col.5.

9 'By the way', *Northern Chronicle and General Advertiser for the North of Scotland*, 27 May 1885, p. col.1.

10 C.M. Watson, *The Life of Major-General Sir Charles Wilson*, p.348.

11 One example of the local support reads, 'The unfair criticisms of which Sir CHARLES has been made the subject must have been read with pain by some Cheltonians, who remember him as a young fellow townsman and a student of Cheltenham College. But we have no fear that in the end they will do him any harm'. See 'Sir Chas. Wilson's Vindication', *Cheltenham Examiner*, 27 May 1885, p.4, col.5.

12 'Notes and Comments', *Gloucestershire Echo*, 8 May 1885, p.2, col.5.

13 Ibid.

14 Lord Cavendish of Keighley (also known as Spencer Compton Cavendish, 8th Duke of Devonshire) (1833-1908), served as Secretary of State for War from 1882 to 1885. He also persuaded Gladstone to establish the Gordon Relief Expedition.

15 'Sir Charles Wilson and the Fall of Khartoum', *Morning Post*, 28 May 1885, p.5, col. 7.

16 'Notes and Comments', *Gloucestershire Echo*, 8 May 1885, p.2, cols.4-5.

17 *Cheltenham Chronicle*, 21 July 1885, p.4, col.5.

18 See, for example, the following extract: 'I thought at the time that, if we had reached Khartum before it fell, the presence of two armed steamers with a small detachment of British soldiers (twenty) might have turned the scale in General Gordon's favour. The fuller knowledge which I now possess of the condition of the garrison, and of the determination of the Mahdi to attack Khartum before the English arrived, leads me to believe that if the steamers had left Gubat a week earlier, the result would have been the same; and that even if it had been possible for them to have reached Khartum on the 25th January, their presence would not have averted the fall of the city.' See Charles W. Wilson, *From Korti to Khartum; a journal of the desert march from Korti to Gubat and of the ascent of the Nile in General Gordon's steamers*, William Blackwood and Sons, 1886, p.vi-vii.

19 C.M. Watson, *The Life of Major-General Sir Charles Wilson*, John Murray, 1909.

20 Ibid., p.355.

21 *ML*, p.342.

Notes to Chapter 12

1 See B.A., 'An officer of health wanted', *Cheltenham Examiner*, 16 October 1867, p.8, cols.4-5. Note: although this letter is signed 'B.A.', it seems likely that this was a pseudonym used by ETW on this occasion given that the content of this letter accords with the letter he claims to have written in October 1867 in his autobiographical notes (see *ML*, p.121).

2 The first Medical Officer of Health was appointed following the Public Health Act (sanitary 1846), which led to the role being established in Liverpool. However, it was not until the Public Health Acts of 1872 and 1875 that it became a statutory duty for districts to appoint medical officers.

3 See *Cheltenham Examiner*, 17 December 1884, p.4, col.6.

4 *ML*, p.184.

5   Ibid., p.186.

6   In 2012, a blue plaque commemorating Ted Wilson was installed at *The Crippetts*, on the house now called Hillcrest.

7   See *Cheltenham Chronicle*, 30 July 1887, p.5, col.4.

8   In 1888 Mary started offering Cheltenham residents twice-daily deliveries of milk. See 'New milk', *Cheltenham Looker-On*, 23 June 1888, p.2, col.3.

9   During the summer of 1898 ETW noted that '... the [Dexter] cows she bought got too fat, and all ended in beef instead of milk'. See *ML*, p.264.

10 *ML*, p.189.

11 Ibid., p.279.

12 Ibid., p.193.

13 The paper was also reproduced in the local press. See 'Cheltenham Natural Science Society', *Cheltenham Examiner*, 24 December 1884, p.2, cols.2-5.

14 The case, which referred to Mary A. Wilson as 'M. A. W.' and Alice M. W. Ingram as 'A. I.' was published by the Society for Psychical Research: 'The following case, received in September, 1885, from Mrs. Wilson, of Westal, Cheltenham, is interesting as an apparent victory of "thought-reading" over "muscle-reading". A group of five "willers" one of whom was in contact with the would-be percipient, were to concentrate their minds on the desire that the latter should sit down to the piano and strike the middle C. Had she done so, the result would have been worth little; but this was what happened: "When A. I. entered blindfolded - her hand in the hand of B, held over the forehead - M. A. W. was possessed with the desire to will her, without bodily contact, to come to her and give her a kiss on the forehead, and she at once exerted (unknown to the others) all her will to achieve this object. A. I. came slowly up to M. A. W., till she stood quite close, touching her, and commenced bending down towards her, when M. A. W., thinking it was hardly fair to succeed against the other 'willers', tried to reverse her will, and with intense effort willed A. I. to turn away and not give the intended kiss. Slowly A. I. raised her head, stood a moment still, then turned in another direction towards the piano, but not near it, and sat down in an armchair. A few seconds after she said: 'I can't feel any impression now, nor any wish to do anything.' She was released from her bandage and questioned as to her feelings. 'Did you get any impression of what you had to do? What did you feel?' She replied: 'I had a distinct feeling that I had to go and kiss M. A. W. on the forehead; but when I came up to someone and bent down to do it, I was sensible of a strong feeling that I was not to do it - and could not do it; and after that I could get no impression whatever.' See Edmund Gurney, *Frederic William Henry Myers, and Frank Podmore, Phantasms of the Living*, vol. 1, Rooms of the Society for Psychical Research, 1886, p.82.

15 Examples of talks given by ETW to Friends in Council around this time included one on the 'Duality of the mind' (1885) and 'Hypnotism' (1888).

16 E.T. Wilson, 'The mind's eye', *Cheltenham Natural Science Society*: 1884, p.187.

17 Ibid., p.188.

18 See 'The mechanism of speech', *Cheltenham Examiner*, 24 November 1886,

p.3, cols.2-4.

19 E.T. Wilson, 'The mind's eye', p.188.

20 *ML*, p.175.

21 Ibid.

22 See *Cheltenham Examiner*, 24 February 1886, p.4, col.6.

23 *ML*, p.191.

24 Ibid.

25 See, for example, 'The Hospital Board's defence', *Cheltenham Examiner*, 24 March 1886, p.4, cols. 6-7.

26 *ML*, p.191.

27 Ibid., p.193.

Notes to Chapter 13

1 Edward T. Wilson, 'The Attractions of Cheltenham', *Cheltenham Examiner*, 20 January 1886, p.8, col.4.

2 Ibid.

3 *ML*, p.169.

4 'The Montpellier Gardens as a local Jubilee memorial', *Cheltenham Chronicle*, 19 March 1887, p.5, cols.4-5.

5 See advertisement in *Cheltenham Chronicle*, 1 May 1886, p.4, col.1.

6 See Edward T. Wilson, 'The future of Cheltenham', 27 January 1892, *Cheltenham Examiner*, p.4, col.5; E. T. Wilson ,'The future of Cheltenham', 3 February 1892, *Cheltenham Examiner*, p.4, col.7; Edward T. Wilson, 'The future of Cheltenham – III', 10 February 1892, *Cheltenham Examiner*, p.4, col.7; 'The future of Cheltenham – IV', 17 February 1892, *Cheltenham Examiner*, p.4, col.6.

7 Weber's reputation as an authority on the spas and mineral waters of Europe was later gained through publication of a definitive book on the subject entitled *The Spas and Mineral Waters of Europe, with notes on balneo-therapeutic management in various diseases and morbid conditions* (Smith, Elder & Co., 1896).

8 See 'Cheltenham as a spa', *Cheltenham Examiner*, 30 March 1892, p.3, cols.1-4; and 'The revival of the Cheltenham spa', *Gloucestershire Echo*, 25 March 1892, p.3, cols.4-7.

9 'The revival of the Cheltenham spa', *Gloucestershire Echo*, 25 March 1892, p.3, cols.4-7.

10 Ibid.

11 Ibid.

12 W., 'A nineteenth century spa. Harrogate – I', *Cheltenham Examiner*, 9 November 1892, p.8 cols.1-2.

13 *ML*, p.223.

14 See W., 'A nineteenth century spa. Harrogate – I', *Cheltenham Examiner*, 9 November 1892, p.8 cols.1-2; and W., 'A nineteenth century spa. Harrogate – II', *Cheltenham Examiner*, 16 November 1892, p.8, cols.1-2.

15 W., 'A nineteenth century spa. Harrogate – II', p.8.

16 One failed attempt occurred, for example, in April 1894 when the Spa scheme, promoted by the Medical Spa Committee (of which ETW was chair) was opposed by the Rate Payers' Association.

17 ETW commented, 'During August [1896] the scheme for a Kursaal ... came to be identified with the name of Ward Humphreys and that was the cause of its failure'. See *ML*, p.253.

18 'Death of Dr. G. H. Ward Humphreys', *Cheltenham Chronicle*, 12 May 1923, p.6, cols. 3-4.

19 Ibid.

20 Edward T. Wilson, 'A nursing home', *Cheltenham Examiner*, 11 May 1887, p.8, col.5.

21 See 'The Victoria Home', *Gloucestershire Echo*, 16 October 1891, p.3, col.7.

22 'Nursing the sick poor. A sister charity to the hospital', *Cheltenham Examiner*, 25 November 1896, p.2, col.6.

23 See 'The Prince's visit and the record reign', *Cheltenham Examiner*, 17 March 1897, p.3, cols.1-3.

24 'Cheltenham District Nursing Association', *Cheltenham Examiner*, 29 November 1905, p.3, cols.4-5.

25 In 1889, for example, around 30,000 volumes were issued to subscribers. See 'The Cheltenham Library', *Cheltenham Examiner*, 1 May 1889, p.8, col.5.

26 *ML*, p.284.

27 The *Cheltenham Examiner* reported, 'On the morning of the sale two habitues quietly read the newspapers in the news room almost until the chairs they sat in were brought under the hammer'. See 'The passing of a library', *Cheltenham Examiner*, 6 August 1908, p.4, col.6.

28 The school taught a range of technical skills, including geometry, machine construction, building construction, freehand drawing, model drawing, perspective, architectural drawing, anatomical studies, drawing and painting from life, designing for decoration and industrial art, modelling in clay, wood carving.

29 E.T. Wilson, Cheltenham School of Art. 1883. Appeal to the public for assistance to build a School of Art for Cheltenham, p.1.

30 Ibid.

31 See 'Cheltenham School of Art', *Cheltenham Examiner*, 13 April 1887, p.3, cols. 5-6.

32 'The Cheltenham School of Art', *Cheltenham Chronicle*, 29 May 1889, p.6, cols.2-3.

33 'Meeting of Mr Hands' supporters', *Cheltenham Chronicle*, 3 November 1888, p.6, cols.1-2.

34 'The public versus the water policy', *Cheltenham Examiner*, 17 April 1889, p.4, cols.4-5.

35 Although the letter was published in October 1888 verbatim extracts were reproduced in 'The public versus the water policy', *Cheltenham Examiner*, 17 April 1889, p.4, cols.4-5.

36 'The public versus the water policy', p.4.

37 *ML*, p.199.
38 Founded in 1877, membership of the CNSS was restricted to 125 gentlemen. Although women were initially excluded, they were allowed to attend lectures which were held at the Corn Exchange.
39 'Contrasts in Nature', *Cheltenham Chronicle*, 23 November 1889, p.2, cols.5-6.
40 Ibid.
41 'Miss Kate Marsden and the Siberian Lepers', *Gloucestershire Echo*, 25 February 1893, p.3, col.3.
42 *ML*, p.227.
43 Ibid.
44 Ibid., p.205.
45 ETW noted that 'our little darling [Gwladys] was raking vigorously in the best of health and spirits ...'. See *ML*, p.238.
46 ETW expressed some of his grief in a poem he wrote for Mary on 26 November 1894: 'Our Heart's delight, our Earthly pride! / God called our Gwladys to His side'. Cheltenham Borough Council and the Cheltenham Trust/The Wilson Family Collection.
47 E.T. Wilson, *Life of Ted* [early manuscript version], Cheltenham Borough Council and the Cheltenham Trust/The Wilson Family Collection, p.24 (Ref. 2010.23).
48 The Home was situated in Liverpool Place (formerly off High Street, opposite Rodney Road).
49 For further information on the Cheltenham Brigade see Audrey Dingle, 'Cheltenham Gordon Boys Brigade 1890-1925' [https://cheltenhamremembers.org.uk/wp-content/files/2018/06/Gordon-Boys-Brigade-and-WW1.pdf], retrieved 8 April 2020. Dingle notes, 'The aim of the Brigade was to bridge the gap between boys leaving school aged about 14, until they were strong enough and old enough to be a wage earner, and placed as pupils in various trades, become apprentices or work for the railway or the Post Office. They aimed to do this by teaching them to be disciplined, respectful and thrifty, giving the boys a uniform and a daily dinner'.
50 Charly stayed at *Westal* on 26 June, when he also came to inspect the Gordons' Boys.
51 C.M. Watson, *The Life of Major-General Sir Charles Wilson*, John Murray, 1909, p.364.
52 *ML*, p.233.
53 Discovered at 4 a.m., the fire was totally extinguished by 6 a.m. For a detailed report see 'Serious fire in Cheltenham', *Cheltenham Chronicle*, 16 December 1893, p.3, col.6.
54 *ML*, p.220.

Notes to Chapter 14

1   The lecture was published in two parts in the *Cheltenham Examiner*. See 'Natural Science Society. Inaugural address by Dr. E. T. Wilson, 'Man and the extinction of species', *Cheltenham Examiner*, 31 October 1894, p.6, cols.2-

3; and 'Natural Science Society. Inaugural address by Dr. E. T. Wilson, 'Man and the extinction of species', *Cheltenham Examiner*, 7 November 1894, p.6, cols.5-6.

2 'Natural Science Society. Inaugural address by Dr. E. T. Wilson, 'Man and the extinction of species', *Cheltenham Examiner*, 31 October 1894, p.6, cols.2-3.

3 Ibid.

4 Ibid.

5 For example, ETW presented a paper on 'The morality of field sports' to the Friends in Council in 1871.

6 *ML*, p.6.

7 'Man and the extinction of species', p.6.

8 Clive Phillipps-Wolley *et al*, *Big Game Shooting*, vol. 2 (Longmans, Green, and Co., 1894), p.71.

9 'Man and the extinction of species', p.6.

10 The society was formed in 1885 and named in honour of the Selborne pioneering naturalist, Gilbert White.

11 'Man and the extinction of species', p.6.

12 Ibid.

13 Dr E. T. Wilson, *Address by President: Birdnesting*, Cheltenham Natural Science Society, 1896, p.2.

14 Ibid., pp.2-3.

15 Ibid., p.3.

16 Ibid., pp.14-15.

17 Emily Williamson founded the Society for the Protection of Birds, now the Royal Society for the Protection of Birds (RSPB), at her home in Manchester in 1889. ETW commented that it had 'already done much good in a quiet, sensible way'. See Dr E. T. Wilson, Address by President: Birdnesting, p.4.

18 ETW referred to the order dated 3 February 1896, which granted protection to the following birds in Gloucestershire: the goldfinch, the buzzard, the honey buzzard, the kestrel, the merlin, the hobby, the osprey, the kingfisher, the nightingale, the nightjar, the nuthatch, the owls, the sandpiper, the woodpeckers and the wryneck. See Dr E. T. Wilson, *Address by President: Birdnesting*, p.15.

19 Ibid., p.16.

20 Ibid.

21 An example of how ETW's views were disseminated is provided in a summary of ETW's lecture 'Man and the extinction of species' produced for the U.S. journal *Popular Science Monthly*. See William Jay Youmans, ed., *Popular Science Monthly* vol. 48, (November 1895 - April 1896), p.142.

22 Towards the end of March 1912 when Ted lay dying, trapped with Captain Scott in a tent by a howling blizzard at the South Pole, Scott wrote a letter to his 'widow'. In it, inspired by Ted, Scott wrote to Kathleen about his hope for the future of their son, Peter: 'Make the boy interested in natural history if you can; it is better than games; they encourage it at some schools.' (See Robert Falcon Scott, *Scott's Last Expedition* (Smith, Elder & Co.: 1913) vol. 1,

p. 415). These lines perfectly echoed the strongly held views by Ted and his father. From these words sprang the inspiration for important aspects of the conservation movement. Sir Peter Scott grew up to be one of the twentieth century's leading conservationists and the founder of the Wildfowl and Wetlands Trust, which has its headquarters at Slimbridge in Gloucestershire, and of the World Wildlife Fund (World Wide Fund for Nature).

Notes to Chapter 15

1   *ML*, p.108.
2   Among the resolutions passed was the following: '... the members of this Society individually feel that they have lost a warm friend, one whose advice and sympathy were always honestly given for the best interests of the Society; and that through the whole period of its existence, the Society has felt the beneficial influence of his personal worth, and of his sound and discriminating judgment ...'. See Committee of the Entomological Society of Philadelphia, *A Memoir of Thomas Bellerby Wilson*, The Entomological Society of Philadelphia, 1865.
3   While ETW records that the resolutions were made by the 'Academy of Sciences of Philadelphia' (see *ML*, pp.108-9) it seems most likely that these are the ones reproduced at the beginning of the following memoir: Committee of the Entomological Society of Philadelphia, *A Memoir of Thomas Bellerby Wilson*, The Entomological Society of Philadelphia, 1865.
4   Ibid., p.35.
5   David O'Connor and Ian Harvey, *Troubled Waters: the great Cheltenham water controversy* (David O'Connor, 2007), p.147.
6   'Severn water', *Cheltenham Examiner*, 31 January 1894, p.8, col.3.
7   *ML*, pp.107-8.
8   ETW noted laconically, '... the less said about it the better'. See *ML*, p.260.
9   See Edward T. Wilson, 'Severn Water', *Cheltenham Examiner*, 16 December 1896, p.8, col. 6.
10 See David O'Connor, p.149.
11 Refers to The Infectious Disease (Notification) Act, 1889.
12 'The "Wilson Block" at the Delancey Hospital. Opening ceremony', *Cheltenham Chronicle*, 27 July 1895, p.2, col.6.
13 'The Delancey Hospital. Opening of the Diphtheria block', *Cheltenham Examiner*, 9 March 1898, p.2, cols.5-7.
14 Ibid.
15 Ibid.
16 'Gloucestershire School of Cookery. Cheltenham Centre opening ceremony', *Cheltenham Chronicle*, 28 January 1899, p.2, cols.6-8.
17 He also commented in a paper read before the CNSS, 'We can all of us recall cases of serious illness, even of death, from the poisonous pork pie, the doubtful sausage, or the cheap tinned meat ... '. See Dr E. T. Wilson, 'Microbes'[second part of an address to a meeting of the Cheltenham Natural Science Society], *Cheltenham Examiner*, 10 November 1897, p.6, cols.5-6.

18 'Cheltenham School of Cookery exhibition and prize giving', *Cheltenham Chronicle*, 1 June 1895, p.6, col.2.

19 *ML*, p.243.

20 Ibid., p.250.

21 *ML*, p.253.

22 See Edward Thomas Wilson, (1832-1918). A single volume of hand-written poems, 1909-1916. Cheltenham Borough Council and the Cheltenham Trust/ The Wilson Family Collection (Ref. 1995.550.176).

23 Ibid., p.265.

24 In his letter to ETW, Ted wrote, 'I am convinced that the sitting still and stuffing and lying out system of cure does kill some people as surely as it cures others. The killing part about it is the lack of occupation, nothing but idle loafing, terribly depressing and demoralizing'. See George Seaver, *Edward Wilson of the Antarctic: naturalist and friend*, (John Murray: 1933), p.55.

25 *ML*, p.272.

Notes to Chapter 16

1   It was reported, 'In 1881 there were sixty-one branches of the C.E.T.S. in the Salisbury diocese, and at the time of [Rathmel's] resignation the number had increased to 215. The numbers of the members in the various sections rose during that time to a very great extent'. See 'Death of Mr. Rathmell [sic] G. Wilson', *Warminster & Westbury journal, and Wilts County Advertiser*, 13 January 1900, p.7, col.6.

2   *ML*, p.276.

3   Ibid., p.277.

4   It is worth noting that on hearing of his nephew's candidacy Charly showed Ted's watercolours to Sir Clements and RGS members.

5   It is interesting to note that ETW provided some case studies for Ted's dissertation on 'Yellow Atrophy of the Liver' which was completed in 1900.

6   Quoted in D.M. Wilson and D.B. Elder, *Cheltenham in Antarctica: the life of Edward Wilson* (Reardon Publishing, 2000), p.51.

7   Later, ETW was probably relieved to hear that although the RRS *Discovery*, the boat in which Ted was first destined to sail to the region, was a wooden three-masted, barque rigged sailing ship, it was also equipped with coal-fired auxiliary steam engines.

8   Later, Scott named Cape Wilson (82°14′S 163°47′E), a headland in Antarctica, after Ted.

9   See in particular Andrew Lyall, 'David Lyall (1817-1895): Botanical explorer of Antarctica, New Zealand, the Arctic and North America', *Linnean* vol. 26, no. 2 (2010), pp. 23-48; and the chapter on Lyall in Ann Lindsay's book, *Seeds of Blood and Beauty: Scottish plant explorers*, Birlinn, 2008.

10 *The Crippetts* was sold to the artist Henry Bowser Wimbush (1858-1943) who later painted a watercolour of the farm.

11 *ML*, p.278.

12 Ibid., p.280.

13 Ibid., p.282.

14 See Alex Shoumatoff, *New Yorker*, 26 April 1982, p. 45.

15 In 1909, she also published *The Old Bureaucrat: a St Petersburg Story*.

16 *ML*, p.283.

17 Ibid., pp.283-4.

18 Indirectly referring to Ted's case, it was reported that ETW said the following: 'He knew a case which had come very near to him, and in which the outdoor treatment had been absolutely successful, and both on private and on public grounds he would recommend it not only to those present but to all whom his words might reach in Cheltenham or in the county'. See 'A Noble Effort. Proposed Sanatorium for Consumptives', *Cheltenham Examiner*, 10 July 1901, p.3, cols.5-7.

19 'A Noble Effort. Proposed Sanatorium for Consumptives', p.3.

20 Ibid.

21 Ibid.

22 This approach proved effective, given the limited medical knowledge and understanding at the time: 'There is no doubt that the open-air treatment was an improvement on the 'cod liver oil era' it replaced and its influence was not challenged until the advent of chemotherapy. The clinicians who introduced the open-air treatment to Britain deserve recognition and credit'. See O. R. McCarthy, 'The key to the sanatoria', *Journal of the Royal Society of Medicine* vol. 94, issue 8 (2001), pp.413-7. McCarthy also concluded: 'An anonymous foreword to the Medical Research Committee Special Report on the Mortality after Sanatorium Treatment (1919) states "The only statistical criterion of the absolute value of sanatorium treatment would be given by a comparison between the rates of mortality of sanatorium patients and those of tuberculosis patients who were similar in age, sex, and economic position, but treated on other lines or untreated.' No such study, or similar statistical comparison was undertaken and it will never be known whether sanatorium treatment was a success or a failure. However, 'Physicians of long and intimate experience of the disease are unanimous in the opinion that the introduction of sanatorium methods has materially improved the outlook for the average consumptive, and that residence in a sanatorium represents the best treatment available at the present time".'

23 *ML*, p.286.

24 ETW was interested to note that the section over which he presided included a paper on 'The Composition and Therapeutic Uses of the Cheltenham Waters' by Dr. Arthur P. Luff, Physician in Charge of Out-patients at St. Mary's Hospital, London. It was later published in the *British Medical Journal*, vol. 2 (issue 2128), 12 October 1901, p.1043.

25 E.T. Wilson, 'Introductory remarks by the President on the value of research in Medicine and Therapeutics' (Sixty-Ninth Annual Meeting of the British Medical Association), *British Medical Journal*, vol. 2 (issue 2128), 12 October 1901, p.1034.

26 Ibid.

27 G. B. Ferguson, 'Sixty-Ninth Annual Meeting of the British Medical Association, Cheltenham, 1901, *British Medical Journal* Volume 1 (Issue 2110), 8 June 1901, pp.1430-3.

28 'B.M.A. Conference in Cheltenham', *Gloucestershire Echo*, 3 August 1901, p.3 col. 2.

29 Ibid.

30 *ML*, p.287.

31 Ibid.

32 The *Gloucestershire Echo* reported, 'If the lecturer's foreign accent sometimes made it a little difficult to follow the story of his adventures and discoveries, ample amends were made by the long series of "dissolving views" of typical bits of Antarctic scenery, of himself, his followers, and their ship (the Southern Cross) amongst "thrilling regions of thick-ribbed ice," and of specimens of the fauna and flora collected See 'Exploring in the Antarctic', *Gloucestershire Echo*, 12 November 1901, p.4, col. 4.

33 *ML*, p.290.

34 On 22 September 1901, Ted recorded: 'After lunch painting a sponge specimen for Murray ...'. See Ann Savours (ed.), *Edward Wilson: Diary of the Discovery Expedition to the Antarctic Regions 1901-1904*, Blandford Press, 1966, p.54.

35 *ML*, p.293.

36 *ML*, p.292.

37 ETW commented that 'his ways were only too well known at the Museum' (See *ML*, p.292).

38 'Cheltenham Town-Hall. Mayoral Banquet', *Gloucestershire Echo*, 2 October 1902, p.3, col.4.

39 For an account of his life, see Percy Scott, *Fifty Years in the Royal Navy*, John Murray, 1919.

40 ETW commented: 'Now with regard to the schools ("Oh!"), the Duke of Wellington had said that "Waterloo was won on the playing field of Eton," a saying which might be made to include all public schools, of which Cheltenham was one (hear, hear)'. As good soldiers were now made in Cheltenham as were made in the Eton of those days (hear, hear)'. See 'Cheltenham Town-Hall. Mayoral Banquet', *Gloucestershire Echo*, 2 October 1902, p.3, col.4.

41 'Cheltenham Town-Hall. Mayoral Banquet', *Gloucestershire Echo*, 2 October 1902, p.3, col.4.

42 Ibid.

43 E.T. Wilson, 'Antarctica', *Cheltenham Natural Science Society*, 1902, p.1. (Note: also published as Dr. E.T. Wilson, 'Antarctica', *Cheltenham Examiner*, 29 October 1902, p.3, cols. 6-7, and Dr. E.T. Wilson, 'Antarctica', *Cheltenham Examiner*, 5 November 1902, p.6, cols.4-6).

44 Ibid., p.2

45 Ibid., p.1.

46 *ML*, p.298.

47 See Ann Savours (ed.), *Edward Wilson: Diary of the Discovery Expedition to the Antarctic Regions 1901-1904*, Blandford Press, 1966, p.225.

48 'Antarctic Expedition. The first year's work', *London Evening Standard*, 11 June 1903, p.5, col.3.
49 Ibid.
50 Ibid.
51 'The South Pole. Captain Scott's Record', *Daily Telegraph & Courier* (London), 11 June 1903, p.12, col.1.
52 *ML*, p.314.
53 Ibid.
54 Lord Rayleigh was also known as John William Strutt, 3rd Baron Rayleigh of Terling Place.
55 Francis Longe was elected to Friends in Council in April 1871. ETW thought that 'He never could state anything clearly but as one of the FiC he was in his element and kept us all alive in his disputations'. ETW described him as 'the handsomest man of his day at Oxford' but considered him 'a failure' despite becoming private secretary to Mr Goschen and, later, an inspector of the Local Government Board. See *ML*, p.320.
56 *ML*, p.320.
57 Ibid.
58 Ibid., p.322.
59 Ibid., p.323.
60 'Geographical Society's Dinner', *Morning Post*, 17 September 1904, p.3, cols.1-2.
61 Ibid.
62 'A pleasant reception', *Cheltenham Examiner*, 28 September 1904, p.4, col.6.
63 Ibid.
64 *ML*, pp.328.
65 *ML*, pp.328-9.
66 Ibid., p.326.
67 E. T. Wilson, A supposed Roman circus on Cleeve Hill, *Cheltenham Natural Science Society*, 1909, p.2.
68 *ML*, p.342.
69 Ibid.
70 Ibid., p.344.
71 'Dr. E.A.Wilson on Antarctica', *Cheltenham Examiner*, 8 November 1905, p.2, col.6. Ted gave a second lecture a few days later at the Grammar School on the subject of Antarctic Fauna. See 'The Antarctic Fauna. Lecture by Dr. E.A. Wilson', *Gloucestershire Echo*, 9 November 1905, p.3, col.7.

Notes to Chapter 17
1 Site now covered by a 1960s telephone exchange.
2 A former colleague recalled that 'One day he [Ferguson] was making a urinalysis, and was holding a urine glass in one hand when he took his glass of "pick-me-up" from the Dispenser with the other. He was busily chatting; suddenly he stopped talking and all but drank the wrong glass, causing a good deal of merriment to the onlookers'. See G. A. Cardew, *Echoes and reminiscences*

of medical practitioners in Cheltenham of the nineteenth century, Ed. J. Burrow & Co., [1921], p.24.

3 It is thought that *Neige Wilson*, almost certainly inspired by Wilson's Antarctic connections, was based on a French dessert, most likely *œufs à la neige* ('eggs in snow') or *île flottante* ('floating island'). Both desserts comprise meringues: while *île flottante* is usually prepared with one large meringue, smaller scoops of meringue are used for *œufs à la neige*.

4 The description of the dinner is given in 'Sayings and Doings of Cheltenham', *Cheltenham Looker-On*, 30 June 1906, p.14, col. 1.

5 The *Cheltenham Examiner* reported ETW's resignation thus, 'We need hardly say to those who know Dr. Wilson and his many activities even outside his profession, that the severance of his connection with the Hospital staff is due to no failure of capacity or energy for the discharge of its duties, and that it does not imply retirement from the practice of his profession. Under the present rules of the Hospital an age limit is imposed upon the medical staff in the interest, less of the institution, perhaps, than that of rising men who may benefit by hospital practice. Though Dr. Wilson is exempt from the operation of this rule he has felt that he ought not to take undue advantage of his exemption, and that the time has come when he should make way for younger men. He would indeed have retired two or three years ago but that certain special considerations in the interest of the Hospital were urged upon him as a reason for the postponement of his action. While his resignation will, as we have said, be received with regret, the motives which have dictated it while delaying its presentation until an opportune moment will alike be appreciated'. See *Cheltenham Examiner*, 30 May 1906, p. 4, col. 7.

6 'The Cheltenham Album', *Gentleman's Magazine*, vol. 98 (October 1828), pp.337-8.

7 'Our early ancestors', *Cheltenham Examiner*, 19 February 1890, p.3, cols. 1-2.

8 Ibid.

9 For a report on the lecture see *Cheltenham Looker-On*, 13 December 1890, p.14, col.2.

10 Dr. E. T. Wilson, *The President's Address read 15 October 1891*, Cheltenham Natural Science Society, 1891.

11 Ibid.

12 In an address to the Field Club at Dean Close School, ETW also spoke about the museum as being 'a place where fellows might go and receive instruction, and not a mere storehouse of curiosities.' See 'Field Club', *Decanian*, vol.3 (no.24), September 1899, p.230.

13 Dr. E. T. Wilson, *The President's Address read 15 October 1891*.

14 Ibid.

15 'A museum for Cheltenham', *Cheltenham Examiner*, 21 October 1891 p.4, cols.4-5.

16 'School of Science', *Cheltenham Chronicle*, 5 December 1891, p.6, col.3.

17 'A museum for Cheltenham', p.4.

18 Ibid.

19 Dr. E. T. Wilson, *The President's Address read 15 October 1891*, Cheltenham Natural Science Society, 1891.

20 Dr. E. T. Wilson, *The President's Address read 15 October 1891*, Cheltenham Natural Science Society, 1891.

21 'Cheltenham Public Museum', *Cheltenham Examiner*, 26 June 1907, p.2, col. 7.

22 'Cheltenham Public Museum', *Cheltenham Examiner*, 19 June 1907, p.8, col. 2.

23 'Cheltenham Public Museum', *Cheltenham Examiner*, 26 June 1907, p.2, col. 7.

24 Ibid.

25 Less than two years later, ETW mourned the loss of Baron de Ferrieres, the town's 'liberal benefactor [who] had given the Art Gallery with its pictures, a window to the Parish Church and the East Window in the College Chapel'. (see *ML*, p.363-4) He added, '...as an MP for Cheltenham he'd not won much confidence, but he was a warm friend ...'. It was typically generous of ETW to praise the baron in this way, given his opposition to vaccination.

26 'Cheltenham Public Museum', *Cheltenham Examiner*, 26 June 1907, p.2, col. 7.

27 A double silver chalice which belonged to ETW is inscribed: 'General Lord Napier of Magdala RE. to Col R. Woodthorpe RE. to Edward T. Wilson M.B. Oxon. FRCP', Cheltenham Borough Council and the Cheltenham Trust/The Wilson Family Collection (Ref. 1995.550.229).

28 ETW refers to a Woodthorpe being one of his patients but, frustratingly, provides no clues for further identification.

29 It is also worth noting that when J. Dalton Woodthorpe donated material to Pitt Rivers in 1916, he wrote, 'I have today sent off a box of saddles &cc, which Miss Wilson wrote to you about which I hope you will find useful for the Museum'. 'Miss Wilson' refers to Ida who donated the bulk of the Woodthorpe drawings in 1929. From information supplied by Dr Chris Morton, Curator of Photograph and Manuscript Collections, Pitt Rivers Museum, in May 2011.

30 Information supplied by Dr Chris Morton, Curator of Photograph and Manuscript Collections, Pitt Rivers Museum, based on an analysis of one of the old picture mounts, which emanates from Cheltenham. It is also thought that ETW 'put some effort into listing the [Woodthorpe] collections and sorting them out, suggesting that they either came to him unsorted, or only partially sorted into the albums which are found at the Pitt Rivers'.

31 *ML*, p.372.

32 Ibid., p.354.

33 It was through Miss Beale that the Ladies' College was transformed, placing as much emphasis on the process of learning, and thereby encouraging independent thinking, as on achieving high levels of educational attainment. During her forty-eight years' tenure as Principal, Miss Beale introduced many reforms, several of which were considered radical at the time.

34 *ML*, p.353.

35 Ibid.

36 ETW commented, '… it was in vain they [the workmen] protested it had to be done otherwise they could not work at the Ladies College'. See *ML*, p.248.

37 *ML*, p.353.

38 Famously, Miss Beale spent several weeks in the sanatorium after she broke a leg while walking on the hill. The sanatorium was rarely used for serious infections and was demolished in 1960.

39 *ML*, p.354.

40 Ibid.

41 Prothero's other work in Cheltenham included the Ladies' College from 1886 to 1895, the chancel of Christ Church, and the Children's Home in Battledown. His work on the Wilson and Diphtheria Blocks of the Delancey Hospital during the 1890s also brought him into close contact with ETW.

42 *ML*, p.355.

43 'Cheltenham Spa, the Inauguration Festivities', *Cheltenham Chronicle*, 23 June 1906, p.6, cols.1-6.

44 Ibid.

45 'The Central Spa', *Cheltenham Examiner*, 20 June 1906, p.8, col. 5-6.

46 The *Cheltenham Examiner* commented, '…the actual Spa has involved comparatively little cost and can hardly be cited as an illustration of municipal enterprise …'. See 'The Central Spa', *Cheltenham Examiner*, 20 June 1906, p.4, col.5.

47 'Cheltenham Spa', *Cheltenham Examiner*, 27 June 1906, p.4, col. 4-5.

48 ETW presented a paper on this subject as President of the Cheltenham Natural Science Society on 21 October 1907.

49 *ML*, p.364

50 Ibid., p.389.

51 Ibid.

52 *ML*, p.364.

53 Dr E. T. Wilson, 'Finger Prints and the Detection of Criminals', *Cheltenham Examiner*, 4 December 1907, p.2, col. 5.

54 See Dr E.T. Wilson, 'The Hand of Man', *Cheltenham Examiner*, 30 October 1907, p.2, col.5.

55 For a report on the lecture, see 'Gen. Baden Powell in Cheltenham. Lecture on Scouting', *Gloucestershire Echo*, 14 January 1908, p.1, col.2.

56 For a report on the lecture, see 'Pre-Historic Egypt', *Cheltenham Examiner*, 5 November 1908, p.8, col. 5.

57 For a report on the lecture, see 'The East Africa Protectorate', *Cheltenham Looker-On*, 1 February 1908, pp.11-12.

58 'Cheltenham Amateur Photographic Society. A Successful Revival', *Gloucestershire Echo*, 29 January 1909, p.3, col. 2.

59 Ibid.

60 ETW's interest in supporting the society may have been partly influenced through the memory of his brother Rathmel who became the Secretary of the Church of England Temperance Society in Salisbury after returning home from Argentina.

61 [Meeting on] 'Alcohol and Life', *Cheltenham Examiner*, 25 November 1909, p.5, col.6.

62 *ML*, pp. 376-7.

63 Ibid., p.374.

64 'Sir Ernest Shackleton on his experiences', *Cheltenham Looker-On*, 4 December 1909, pp.23-4.

65 See *ML*, p.377.

Notes to Chapter 18

1   The Great January Comet of 1910, formally designated C/1910 A1, was one of the brightest comets of the twentieth century.

2   *ML*, p.378.

3   ETW commented that 'its nervous origin seemed decided by the fact of its complete cessation on the departure of the Terra Nova from Cardiff' (see *ML*, p.381).

4   Ted's portrait was exhibited in the Royal Academy in 1910.

5   ETW commented that in September 1913, 'Alf Soord was busy at work on Mary's portrait (a present from my old patient Mr Woodthorpe), which when finished was approved by nearly all the family.' (See *ML*, p.415). Her portrait was completed in 1913.

6   ETW commented, 'This [ETW's] portrait and Ted's were the means of introducing the artist to Mr James Winterbotham whose portrait and that of his wife and brother Sir Henry he subsequently painted with great satisfaction to all'. See *ML*, pp.379-80. This record was used in December 2019 to identify that the work by Soord, dated 1910, held at The Wilson, which was previously entitled 'Portrait of an Unknown Man', was really that of James Winterbotham.

7   Edward T. Wilson, Letter to [E. Bernard Wilson], 17 June [1910], Scott Polar Research Institute Archives, University of Cambridge (Ref. MS 963/4).

8   Ibid.

9   Ibid.

10 *ML*, p.381.

11 ETW commented that he found the telephone 'a useful servant'. See *ML*, p.382.

12 Edward T. Wilson, Letter to [E. Bernard Wilson], 17 June [1910], Scott Polar Research Institute Archives, University of Cambridge (Ref. MS 963/4).

13 The paper was presented on 17 October 1910. ETW described the subject as 'a goodly one which the rising generations were lightly throwing away' (see ML p.386). It was also published in the *Cheltenham Examiner*. See Dr. E.T. Wilson, 'Our Inheritance', *Cheltenham Examiner*, 20 October 1910, p.7, col.3-4; and Dr. E.T. Wilson, 'Our Inheritance (conclusion)', *Cheltenham Examiner*, 27 October 1910, p.6, cols.4-5.

14 Dr. E.T. Wilson, 'Our Inheritance (conclusion)' , p.6.

15 ETW wrote, 'Yet what does history teach us? Through a slow growth, due to selection, exercised by Man himself, an aristocracy of ability has over and

over again been formed and as often wantonly thrown to the winds. It was killed out in Rome with appalling results under the Emperors; it was killed out in large measure in the monasteries and nunneries of the Middle Ages; it was decimated by beheadal or burning in the lurid times of the Tudors in England and in the fierce persecutions of the Inquisition in Spain. The best intellects in Russia are now in Siberian banishment and there are few left at home to govern or direct. The Napoleonic wars made large inroads on the best blood and intellect of Europe. What is to be the experience of the boasted civilisation of the twentieth century? Great Britain was highly favoured throughout the Victorian epoch in the possession of a noble body of men whose aptitude for enterprise and for government and for affairs generally not only created the vast Empire to which we are privileged to succeed, but won the admiration of the civilised world. It was indeed a goodly heritage which was handed down to the generation now reaching its middle age. What has it done with it? The first step affecting it was taken some hundred years ago, when a wave of philanthropy swept over the country. The old laissez faire was deservedly discredited, and every effort was made to preserve human life, whether fit or unfit to take its place in the world, while many valuable lives have been preserved; there can be no doubt that under this protective system the feeble-minded, the criminal, and unsound stock generally have been and are still increasing at an alarming rate, while the upper, middle, and artisan classes are as steadily dwindling in numbers. It is one of the most serious problems of the day, and there are already signs that it is at last awaking the somnolent attention of practical politics'. Ibid.

16 Ibid.
17 Edward Wilson, *Diary of the Terra Nova expedition to the Antarctic 1910-1912* (Blandford Press: 1972), p.118.
18 The lecture was given at Dean Close School on 22 March 1911. See 'The Field Club', *Decanian*, Vol. 7, No. 59 (1911), p.175.
19 16 September 1909.
20 George Seaver, *Edward Wilson of the Antarctic: Naturalist and Friend*, John Murray, 1933, p.182.
21 'The Field Club', *Decanian* Vol. 7, No. 59 (1911), p.175.
22 Ibid., p.176.
23 E.T. Wilson, 'Antarctica', *Cheltenham Natural Science Society*, 1902. Also published as Dr. E.T. Wilson, 'Antarctica', *Cheltenham Examiner*, 29 October 1902, p.3, cols. 6-7, and Dr. E.T. Wilson, 'Antarctica', *Cheltenham Examiner*, 5 November 1902, p.6, cols.4-6.
24 George Seaver, p.245.
25 E.T. Wilson, 'Antarctica', p.9.
26 When Cherry-Garrard became a regular visitor at *Westal*, following Ted's death, ETW commented that they 'had a deeply interesting talk especially upon the Crozier journey' on 23 July 1913. See *ML*, p.411-2. Cherry-Garrard would have shared with ETW the delight he wrote about when they first arrived at the penguin colony in Cape Crozier and started to make scientific

discoveries: 'After indescribable effort and hardship we were witnessing a marvel of the natural world, and we were the first and only men who had ever done so; we had within our grasp material which might prove of the utmost importance to science; we were turning theories into facts with every observation we made ...'. See Apsley Cherry-Garrard, *The Worst Journey in the World*, Picador, 1994 [first published 1922], p.274.

27 Extract from his poem 'Faith. Hope. Love'. See Edward Thomas Wilson, (1832-1918). A single volume of hand-written poems, 1909-1916. Cheltenham Borough Council and the Cheltenham Trust/The Wilson Family Collection (Ref. 1995.550.176).

28 See *ML*, p.395. ETW's description accorded with the local press report: 'Mr. Hucks on Thursday made an easy ascent, and was soon soaring at an altitude of 1,000 ft., then at 1,6110 ft., and remained in the air 19 minutes, flying about twenty miles in three circles, and ultimately safely returned to earth'. See 'Aviation in Cheltenham', *Cheltenham Chronicle*, 7 October 1911, p.2, col.6.

29 See 'British Notes of the Week', *Flight Magazine*, (October 1911), p.894. Despite the apparent danger, this exhibition flight for the Cheltenham Collegians also ended safely 'as [Hucks] made a graceful *vol plané* landing without damage in a neighbouring field to the Whaddon Farm, where his hangar was erected'. Another hazardous moment at Cheltenham, following a forced landing, was 'when he ploughed up yards of cabbages with his skids until eventually a wheel came off and moving forward broke the airscrew'. See Amina Chatwin and Steve Osmond, 'Cheltenham and the men in their flying machines', *Cheltenham Local History Society Journal* 30 (2014), p.57.

30 Along with Shackleton, Jameson Adams and Frank Wild, Marshall was one of the four men who reached Farthest South at 88°23'S 162°00'E on 9 January 1909.

31 *ML*, p.397.

32 Ibid., pp.397-8.

33 Ibid., p.400.

34 'A keen controversialist, Dr. Bond took an especial interest in the question of vaccination, the cause of which he was ready at all times and upon all occasions to champion, and was prominently associated with the formation of the Jenner Society, of which he was the Honorary Secretary'. See *Gloucester Citizen*, 6 December 1911, p.2, col.6.

35 *ML*, p.400.

36 Edward Wilson, *Diary of the Terra Nova expedition to the Antarctic 1910-1912*, p.232.

37 Ibid.

38 *ML*, p.400. ETW described Hart as 'a grand man and much more than a soldier, for he thinks'.

39 Edward T. Wilson, Letter to Reginald Smith, 14 February 1913, Scott Polar Research Institute Archives, University of Cambridge (Ref. MS 559/147/2).

40 E.T. Wilson, 'Antarctica', p.12.

41 See Hugh S. Torrens and Michael A. Taylor, 'Geological collectors and museums in Cheltenham 1810-1988: a case history and its lessons', *Geological Curator* vol.5 (issue 2 for 1988), p.192.

42 Ibid.

43 Ibid.

44 E.T. Wilson, Extracts of letters, on a single sheet of paper, copied by Edward Thomas Wilson (1832-1918) from Edward Wilson of the Antarctic (1872-1912) to his parents, Cheltenham Borough Council and the Cheltenham Trust/The Wilson Family Collection (Ref. 1995.550.104a).

45 Telegram from Ory to the family at Westal, 3 April 1912, Cheltenham Borough Council and the Cheltenham Trust/The Wilson Family Collection (Ref. 2010.36).

46 In reality they were 169 miles from the Pole.

47 'South Polar Exploration', *Cheltenham Examiner*, 4 April 1912, p.4, cols 3-4.

48 *ML,* p.401.

49 ETW commented that he persuaded Witts to leave his collection of flints from the Cotswolds to the town museum where, with other collections, 'it forms one of the most attractive features' (see *ML,* p.405).

50 Edward T. Wilson, Letter to Reginald Smith, 16 June 1912, Scott Polar Research Institute Archives, University of Cambridge (Ref. MS 559/147/1).

51 The walk took place on 20 July 1912. See 'Botany of Combe Hill and Wainlode', *Cheltenham Examiner*, 25 July 1912, p.5, col.6. Despite the conditions, this is the list of specimens they discovered and in the order in which they found them: Great water dock (Rumen hydrolapathum); Bullrushes or reed-mace (Typha Latifolia); Blue skull-cap (Scutellaria gatericulata); Creeping Jenny (Lysimachia nummularia); 2 Water-dropworts (Ananthe phellandrium & A. Fistulosa); Purple loose-strife (Lythrum saliearia); Yellow loose-strife (Lysimachia vulgaris); Tufted vetch (Vicia cracca); Flowering rush (Butomus umbellatus); Water-plantain (Alisma plantago); Arrow-head (Sagittaria sagiltifolia); Amphibious bistort (Polygonum amphibium); Frog-bit (Hydrocharis Morsusrancae); 2 forms of Starwort (Callitriche); Water crowfoot (Ranunculus heterophyllus); One of the pondweeds (Polamogeton pictinatus); 2 species of buck-weed (Lemma gibba & L. Minor); Fetid chara (Chara foetida); Marsh woundwort (Stachys palustris); Blur-reed (Sparganium ramosum); Horned pondweed (Zannichellia palustris); Large leaved form of the Yellow Medow-rue (Thalictum flavum); Strawberry headed clover (Trifolium fragiferum); Meadow-cranes-bill (Geranium pratense); Great Burnet (Sanguiosorba officinalis); Black mustard (Brassica nigra); 3 members of the watercress family (Nasturtium sylvestre, N.terrestre, N. Amphidium); 2 more pondweeds (Polamogeton perfiliatum, P. Flabellatum); Water speedwell (Veronica anagallis); Marsh cudweed (Graphalium uliginosum).

52 British Antarctic Expedition Pictures, *Pall Mall Gazette* 24 August 1912, p.9, col. 3.

53 *ML,* p.403.

54 Edward Wilson, *Diary of the Terra Nova expedition to the Antarctic 1910-1912*

(Blandford Press: 1972), p.174.
55 *Cheltenham Looker-On*, 7 December 1912, p.7.
56 *ML*, p.406-7.
57 E.T. Wilson, 'Antarctica', p.14.
58 'The Field Club', *Decanian*, Vol. 7, No. 61 (1912), pp. 276-280.
59 Ibid., p.280.
60 *ML*, p.408.
61 Ibid.
62 Ibid., p.409.
63 Ibid.
64 'Wilson Memorial Fund. Expressions of Sympathy', *Cheltenham Looker-On*, 22 February 1913, [n.p.], col.2.
65 Edward T. Wilson, Letter to Reginald Smith, 14 February 1913, Scott Polar Research Institute Archives, University of Cambridge (Ref. MS 559/147/2).
66 Max Jones, *The Last Great Quest: Captain Scott's Antarctic Sacrifice*, Oxford University Press, 2003, p.133.
67 W, 'Captain Scott and His Companions', *The Times*, 19 February, 1913, No. 40139, p.5, col.3.
68 The correct date should have been recorded as 29 March 1912.
69 *ML*, p.409.
70 Ibid.
71 'The South Pole Disaster: Proposed Memorial to Dr. Adrian Wilson', *Cheltenham Examiner*, 6 March 1913, p.3, col. 1.
72 'Correspondence', *Cheltenham Looker-On*, 31 January 1914, p.21, col.1.
73 'The South Pole Disaster: Proposed Memorial to Dr. Adrian Wilson', p.3.
74 The *Cheltenham Chronicle* reported that the local M.P. James T. Agg-Gardner described the decision as follows: 'The question of the form the [Wilson] memorial should take then arose. There were naturally differences of opinion – "many men, many opinions" - and many interesting and ingenious suggestions were offered. In the end we thought the best solution of the problem would be to consult the feelings of the family. We took this course, and were at once relieved from the anxieties of decision by the kindness and wisdom of Dr. Wilson. He recommended a bronze statue as being the most suitable and acceptable form of memorial, and rendered his recommendation still more attractive by a suggestion that Lady Scott might be persuaded to undertake the execution of the work, and a promise to use his personal endeavours to obtain her consent'. See 'A Cheltenham Hero. Wilson Statue Unveiled', *Cheltenham Chronicle*, 11 July 1914, p.8, cols. 6-8.
75 'The South Pole Disaster: Proposed Memorial to Dr. Adrian Wilson', p.3.
76 The *Cheltenham Chronicle* reported: 'Out of friendship for the family of Dr. Wilson, Lady Scott, who enjoys a high reputation as an artist, offered to undertake the designing of the statue of her husband's old comrade as a labour of love. The [Wilson] Memorial Committee, however, did not feel able to accept this generous offer in full, but arranged with Lady Scott to undertake the work at considerably less than her usual fee for such a work'.

See 'A Cheltenham Hero. Wilson Statue Unveiled', *Cheltenham Chronicle*, 11 July 1914, p.8, cols. 6-8.

77 The poem is dated 10 April 1913. See Dr Edward Thomas Wilson, Poems by Edward Thomas Wilson, 1909-1916, Cheltenham Borough Council and the Cheltenham Trust/The Wilson Family Collection (Ref. 1995.550.176).

78 The poem is dated 18 April 1913. See Dr Edward Thomas Wilson, Poems by Edward Thomas Wilson, 1909-1916, Cheltenham Borough Council and the Cheltenham Trust/The Wilson Family Collection (Ref. 1995.550.176).

79 Ibid.

80 ETW noted that 'He [Debenham] and Cherry-Garrard are our favourites among the Antarctics and the article in the Caian by the former show at once his literary ability and his devotion to Ted'. See *ML*, p.415.

81 ETW notes that on 23 April 1913, 'Dr Atkinson came for the night. He being one of the rescue party who found the tent had much to tell and we were glad of the opportunity for hearing things first hand and direct'. See *ML*, p.410.

82 Ibid., p.411.

83 Quoted in Katherine MacInnes, *Woman with the Iceberg Eyes: Oriana F. Wilson*, The History Press, 2019, p.205.

84 *ML*, p.412.

85 'A letter was read from [ETW as] the Hon. Secretary of the Delancey Hospital, stating that the Trustees had decided that, owing to changing conditions, it is no longer possible to carry on the Hospital in the manner originally intended by the Founders, and that they had therefore approached the Charity Commissioners, who expressed their willingness to prepare and sanction a scheme for vesting the management of the Hospital in a Board of representatives of the public bodies in Cheltenham and the neighbourhood who are under an obligation to provide accommodation for the treatment of infectious diseases - and possibly for tuberculous patients - and who would be prepared to contribute to the cost of the maintenance of the Hospital'. See 'Delancey Hospital', *Cheltenham Examiner*, 11 September 1913, p.8, col.6.

86 'The Delancey Hospital Scheme', *Cheltenham Examiner*, 16 October 1913, p.6, col.4.

87 *ML.*, p.412.

88 Edward T. Wilson, *The Long-Barrow Men of the Cotswolds*, Cheltenham Natural Science Society, 1913, p.3.

89 Ibid., p.10.

90 Later, ETW donated a cast of the Piltdown Skull to Bristol Museum. Since then, it has been transferred to The Wilson (Cheltenham Art Gallery and Museum).

91 Fluorine tests in 1949 showed that the Piltdown skull was only 50,000 years old. This discounted the theory that it could be the 'missing link' between humans and apes because, by then, humans had already developed into Homo Sapiens. Additional tests revealed the use of filing tools and artificial staining methods to distort the evidence further. See 'Piltdown Man' at https://www.nhm.ac.uk/our-science/departments-and-staff/library-and-archives/

collections/piltdown-man.html (retrieved 27 December 2019).

92 *ML*, p.417.

93 Such was the popularity of this exhibition that the opening hours had to be extended until 10 o'clock at night to cope with the huge number of visitors.

94 *ML*, p.417.

95 During a visit to London on 9 December 1912, when he saw an exhibition on the Antarctic and the Piltdown skull at the Natural History Museum and then visited an exhibition of Ponting's photographs, ETW also recorded that 'We also had time for a view of Lady Scotts [sic] statue of Ted, a noble figure ...'. See *ML*, p.416.

96 'A Cheltenham Hero. Wilson Statue Unveiled', *Cheltenham Chronicle*, 11 July 1914, p.8, cols. 6-8.

97 *ML*, p.418.

98 Agg-Gardner '[wished to] 'express the regret of the [Town Council] committee that we are meeting to-day without the presence of one of our members who took great interest in this memorial, both as a personal friend of Dr. Wilson, and also as one who was a lover of Art. I refer to the late Mr. James Winterbotham. We deeply deplore his loss, and we all miss to-day his pleasant presence, his captivating eloquence, and the sunshine of that genial humour, which, as has been said of summer lightning, brightens but does not burn'. 'A Cheltenham Hero. Wilson Statue Unveiled', *Cheltenham Chronicle*, 11 July 1914, p.8, cols. 6-8.

99 ETW commented: 'There was a good deal of entertaining and standing about so not surprising that a sharp attack came on'. See *ML*, p.419.

100 Letter from E.T. Wilson to Apsley Cherry-Garrard, 14 July 1914. Scott Polar Research Institute Archives, University of Cambridge (Ref. MS 1330/5).

101 Ibid.

Notes to Chapter 19

1 *ML*, p. 420.

2 Lothar Kettenacker, ed., *The Legacies of Two World Wars: European Societies in the Twentieth Century, Torsten Riotte*, (Berghahn Books, 2011) pp. 58-9.

3 Letter from E. Bernard Wilson to Edward Thomas Wilson, 19 August 1914, Cheltenham Borough Council and the Cheltenham Trust/The Wilson Family Collection (Ref. 1995.550.77).

4 Jilly Cooper, *Animals in war*, (Corgi: 1984), p.12.

5 E.T. Wilson, *Man under evolution*, Cheltenham Natural Science Society, 1898, p. 12.

6 Ibid., p. 13.

7 Ibid.

8 *ML*, p.419.

9 Letter from E. Bernard Wilson to Edward Thomas Wilson, 18 October 1914, Cheltenham Borough Council and the Cheltenham Trust/The Wilson Family Collection (Ref. 1995.550.77).

10 E.T. Wilson, *Man under evolution*, Cheltenham Natural Science Society, 1898,

p.10.

11   Francis Cox, *The First World War: Disease, the Only Victor* [transcript of a lecture given on 10 March 2014 at the Museum of London], Gresham College, 1984, p.2.

12   Letter from E. Bernard Wilson to Edward Thomas Wilson, 18 October 1914, Cheltenham Borough Council and the Cheltenham Trust/The Wilson Family Collection (Ref. 1995.550.77).

13   *ML*, p.287.

14   Cox, p.3. Osler's arguments that vaccination against typhoid would reduce mortality by half ensured that 97% of troops were vaccinated.

15   Cholera belts, made of flannel or knitted wool, were worn around the abdomen before wearing a shirt and were once thought to be a preventive measure against cholera and dysentery caused by the chilling of the abdomen. For further information see E.T. Renbourn, 'The history of the flannel binder and cholera belt', *Medical History* 1 (3) (1957), pp. 211–225. This quotes the official medical history of the First World War which noted that 'there was a unanimity of opinion that body bands did not contribute either to comfort, warmth or health, and soldiers themselves disliked wearing bands as they harboured vermin'.

16   Bernard was stationed then at the Witley Military Camp set up on Witley Common near Godalming, Surrey.

17   Letter from E. Bernard Wilson to Edward Thomas Wilson, 16 December 1914, Cheltenham Borough Council and the Cheltenham Trust/The Wilson Family Collection (Ref. 1995.550.77).

18   Letter from Mary Rendall (née Wilson) to Edward Thomas Wilson, 12 February 1915, Cheltenham Borough Council and the Cheltenham Trust/The Wilson Family Collection (Ref. 1995.550.64).

19   Letter from E. Bernard Wilson to Mary Agnes Wilson, 21 February 1916, Cheltenham Borough Council and the Cheltenham Trust/The Wilson Family Collection (Ref. 1995.550.77).

20   The portrait of Ted was painted by Hugh Rivière, with the exception of the husky dogs, which were painted by Hugh's father, Briton, who was educated at Cheltenham College where his father, William Rivière, was drawing master between 1850 and 1858.

21   Recording of an interview between Dr David Wilson and Peter Rendall, together with his sister Betty Rendall, at Chippings, 155 The Hill, Burford on 21 September 1996. Cheltenham Borough Council and the Cheltenham Trust/The Wilson Family Collection.

22   Michael Bliss, *William Osler: A Life in Medicine*, (Oxford University Press, 1999), p.413.

23   Harvey Cushing, *The Life of Sir William Osler*, vol. 2, (Oxford University Press, 1940), pp.1166-7.

24   In his sixties, it is worth noting that Osler often bought medical manuscripts from the vast library created by Sir Thomas Phillipps at Thirlestaine House in Cheltenham. See John Cule, 'Sir William Osler and his Welsh connections',

Postgraduate Medical Journal 64 (1988), p.573.

25 William Osler, *Bibliotheca Osleriana: a catalogue of books illustrating the history of medicine and science*, McGill-Queen's University Press, 1969, p.687. The index entry is 7633.

26 Note: permission to quote from 'A Retrospect' was granted by Dr David Wilson on behalf of the Wilson family.

27 *ML*, p.435.

28 Ibid., p.438.

29 Ibid.

30 Today, the portrait hangs in the College's Common Room.

31 'Dr. Edward Adrian Wilson Cheltenham College memorial unveiled', *Cheltenham Chronicle*, 25 September 1915, p.7, col.4.

32 *ML*, p.433.

33 Ibid.

34 Ibid., p.422.

35 One of the stanzas of the poem read: 'God of Battles hear us / Hear us while we pray / Guard and guide our dear ones / On this holy day.'

36 Letter from E. Bernard Wilson to Edward Thomas Wilson, 13 February 1916, Cheltenham Borough Council and the Cheltenham Trust/The Wilson Family Collection (Ref. 1995.550.77).

37 E.T. Wilson, *Man under evolution*, Cheltenham Natural Science Society, 1898, p. 13.

38 Letter from E. Bernard Wilson to Edward Thomas Wilson, 6 February 1916, Cheltenham Borough Council and the Cheltenham Trust/The Wilson Family Collection (Ref. 1995.550.77).

39 Ibid.

40 Minutes of the Friends in Council, see report of 464th meeting on 1 February 1916.

41 Letter from E. Bernard Wilson to Edward Thomas Wilson, 13 February 1916, Cheltenham Borough Council and the Cheltenham Trust/The Wilson Family Collection (Ref. 1995.550.77).

42 Ibid.

43 Letter from E. Bernard Wilson to Edward Thomas Wilson and Mary Agnes Wilson, 28 February 1916, Cheltenham Borough Council and the Cheltenham Trust/The Wilson Family Collection (Ref. 1995.550.77).

44 Ibid.

45 Letter from E. Bernard Wilson to Edward Thomas Wilson and Mary Agnes Wilson, 20 March 1916, Cheltenham Borough Council and the Cheltenham Trust/The Wilson Family Collection (Ref. 1995.550.77).

46 Letter from E. Bernard Wilson to Edward Thomas Wilson and Mary Agnes Wilson, 24 March 1916, Cheltenham Borough Council and the Cheltenham Trust/The Wilson Family Collection (Ref. 1995.550.77).

47 Letter from E. Bernard Wilson to Mary Agnes Wilson, 7 April 1916, Cheltenham Borough Council and the Cheltenham Trust/The Wilson Family Collection (Ref. 1995.550.77).

48 Letter from E. Bernard Wilson to Edward Thomas Wilson, 15 April 1916, Cheltenham Borough Council and the Cheltenham Trust/The Wilson Family Collection (Ref. 1995.550.77).

49 Ibid.

50 Letter from E. Bernard Wilson to Edward Thomas Wilson and Mary Agnes Wilson, 18 April 1916, Cheltenham Borough Council and the Cheltenham Trust/The Wilson Family Collection (Ref. 1995.550.77).

51 *Cheltenham Looker-On*, 22 April 1916, p.11, col.2.

52 Letter from E. Bernard Wilson to Edward Thomas Wilson and Mary Agnes Wilson, 12 April 1916, Cheltenham Borough Council and the Cheltenham Trust/The Wilson Family Collection (Ref. 1995.550.77).

53 Ibid.

54 Letter from E. Bernard Wilson to Edward Thomas Wilson, 23 July 1916 (Ref. 1995.550.77); and Letter from E. Bernard Wilson to Edward Thomas Wilson, 4 August 1916, Cheltenham Borough Council and the Cheltenham Trust/The Wilson Family Collection (Ref. 1995.550.77).

55 Letter from E. Bernard Wilson to Edward Thomas Wilson, 26 July 1916, Cheltenham Borough Council and the Cheltenham Trust/The Wilson Family Collection (Ref. 1995.550.77).

56 Letter from E. Bernard Wilson to Edward Thomas Wilson, 21 August 1916, Cheltenham Borough Council and the Cheltenham Trust/The Wilson Family Collection (Ref. 1995.550.77).

57 Letter from E. Bernard Wilson to Edward Thomas Wilson, 1 September 1916, Cheltenham Borough Council and the Cheltenham Trust/The Wilson Family Collection (Ref. 1995.550.77).

58 Letter from E. Bernard Wilson to Mary Agnes Wilson, 21 September 1916, Cheltenham Borough Council and the Cheltenham Trust/The Wilson Family Collection (Ref. 1995.550.77).

59 Turtle Bunbury, 'The Whishaws: From Rudheath to Russia, 2006' http://www.turtlebunbury.com/history/history_family/hist_family_whishaw.html [retrieved 2 November 2019].

60 Letter from E. Bernard Wilson to Edward Thomas Wilson, 22 April 1917, Cheltenham Borough Council and the Cheltenham Trust/The Wilson Family Collection (Ref. 1995.550.77).

61 Letter from E. Bernard Wilson to Edward Thomas Wilson, 14 May 1917, Cheltenham Borough Council and the Cheltenham Trust/The Wilson Family Collection (Ref. 1995.550.77).

62 Letter from E. Bernard Wilson to Edward Thomas Wilson, 31 December 1917, Cheltenham Borough Council and the Cheltenham Trust/The Wilson Family Collection (Ref. 1995.550.77).

63 Letter from E. Bernard Wilson to Edward Thomas Wilson, 29 March 1918, Cheltenham Borough Council and the Cheltenham Trust/The Wilson Family Collection (Ref. 1995.550.77).

64 For a full report see 'The late Dr. E.T. Wilson. Funeral at Leckhampton', *Gloucestershire Echo*, 23 April 1918, p.4 col.2.

65 Letter from E. Bernard Wilson to Mary Agnes Wilson, 25 April 1918, Cheltenham Borough Council and the Cheltenham Trust/The Wilson Family Collection (Ref. 1995.550.77).

66 Ibid.

67 Letter from E. Bernard Wilson to Mary Agnes Wilson, 11 November 1918, Cheltenham Borough Council and the Cheltenham Trust/The Wilson Family Collection (Ref. 1995.550.77).

Notes to Chapter 20

1   'Obituary. Dr. E.T. Wilson, F.R.C.P.', *Cheltenham Looker-On*, 27 April 1918, p.11, cols.1-2.

2   Ibid.

3   Ibid.

4   'Death of Dr. E.T. Wilson', *Gloucestershire Echo*, 20 April 1918, p.4, col.4.

5   It was not until the 1860s that the idea of an 'isolation hospital' had started to develop. See Matthew Newsom Kerr, *Contagion, Isolation, and Biopolitics in Victorian London*, (Springer Nature, 2018), p.34.

6   See, for example, the article published by the *Spectator* on 15 May 2020 entitled Let's bring back Britain's fever hospitals by Professor Carl Heneghan and Tom Jefferson, two experts from University of Oxford. [https://www.spectator.co.uk/article/Lets-bring-back-Britains-fever-hospitals, retrieved 21 June 2021].

7   J. Francis Sutherland, 'Necessity for and Location of Contagious and Infectious Hospitals', *Glasgow Medical Journal* vol. 16 (September 1881), p.178. Previously, ETW had promoted his ideas through an article, 'Isolation as a means of arresting epidemic disease', published in *Practitioner* in 1879.

8   G. Arthur Cardew, *Echoes and Reminiscences of Medical Practitioners in Cheltenham of the Nineteenth Century* (Ed. J. Burrow & Co. Ltd., 1930), p.18.

9   'Death of Dr. E.T. Wilson', *Gloucestershire Echo*, 20 April 1918, p.4, col.4.

10 Ibid.

11 'Obituary. Dr. E.T. Wilson, F.R.C.P.', p.11.

12 While he lists 123 papers at the end of his autobiographical notes (see *ML*, pp.447-54), this is not an exhaustive list.

13 'Death of Dr. E.T. Wilson', p.4.

14 The most significant memoir (still unpublished) that ETW wrote was on Ted's Life. Without this work, Ted's future biographers would have had limited material upon which to draw. See Edward Thomas Wilson of Cheltenham (1832-1918), Edward Adrian Wilson (1872-1912): a memoir by his father. Ref. 1995.550.36.

15 For example, when Ted received ETW's comments on his draft monograph on emperor penguins, he wrote to his father: 'There was not a correction you made that I did not adopt, and you greatly improved the chapters'. See George Seaver, *Edward Wilson of the Antarctic: Naturalist and Friend*, John Murray, 1933, p.146.

16 Ibid., p.143.

17 For details see 'Local wills', *Cheltenham Chronicle*, 10 August 1918, p.2 col.5.

18 Recording of an interview between Dr David Wilson and Peter Rendall, together with his sister Betty, at Chippings, 155 The Hill, Burford on 21 September 1996. Cheltenham Borough Council and the Cheltenham Trust/ The Wilson Family Collection

19 Ibid.

20 Ibid.

Appendices

Appendix 1 – Wilson Family Trees

1   Edward Wilson of Hean Castle (1808-88)

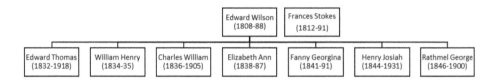

2   Edward Thomas Wilson of Cheltenham (1832-1918)

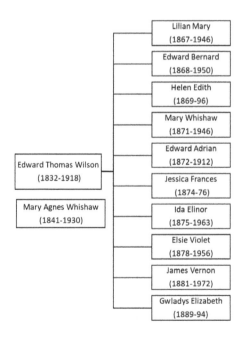

Appendix 2 – Wilson's Method for Photographing Microscopic Objects

This summary is based on ETW's article, 'How to photograph microscopic objects', published in the *Popular Science Review* (vol. 6, 1867, pp. 54-65), and draws on technical insights provided by John White, a member of Cheltenham Camera Club.

Helping to eradicate the need for expensive equipment, ETW maintained that good results could be achieved simply with a good microscope and the modest purchase of other equipment. Some ingenuity and resourcefulness were everything else that was needed. For the photographic chamber, for example, he recommended using 'any type of sitting room'. In his own case, it was the drawing room which he furnished, along with a camera and the necessary chemicals, with a 'candle shaded by a tripod stand of yellow calico ... steady table protected by a stout cloth, a bucket or basin, a jug and a good supply of water'.

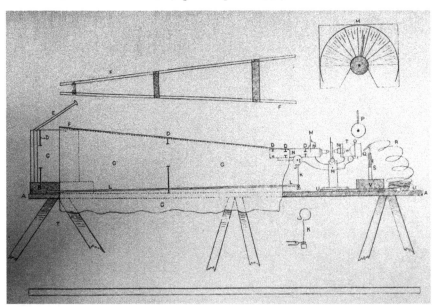

Diagram 1 – The Microscope arranged for Photography (from 'How to photograph microscopic objects')

A – A stout well-seasoned board, 8 feet (Long) x 15 inches (Wide), used as the base-board.
B – A light wooden block used to align the centre of the focusing screen with the axis of the microscope.

C – Focusing box of an ordinary camera.
D – Diaphragms made from tin and coated in black. Once the eye-piece of the microscope had been removed these, together with a tube of black velvet, were introduced into the body of the microscope in place of the draw tube to lightproof the equipment.
E – The Plate Carrier.
F – A triangular framework used to support G.
G – A double fold of cotton velvet used as a blackout.
H – Microscope.
I – Coarse or rack adjustment.
K – Stout brass wire which was attached to the coarse or rack adjustment (I) and used as a lever to make finer focusing adjustments.
L – Long wooden rod, which reaches the focusing screen, used to hold the lever (K) in place.
M – Small dial plate of card which was used to measure the slightest alterations in fine adjustment made to compensate for the differences between the actinic and visual foci.
N – Achromatic condenser (of microscope).
O – Hemispherical drum first used by Reade to assist with centring and adjusting the light.
P – A movable stop of tin with a pinhole aperture.
R – Magnesium wire.
S – Small brass telescope upright regulated by a screw. This was used to direct the magnesium wire (R) downwards at an angle of 45° at the apex of the upright.
T – Supporting trestles.
U – Light block support used to ensure that, when levelled horizontally and accurately centred, a light thrown through the lens of the object glass forms a rounded disc in the centre of the focusing screen at all lengths of the camera.
V – Block adapted to slide on the support.

ETW's method relied on using a good quality lens, either one designed for a microscope or for photography. He stressed the importance of using a small aperture to create the optimum depth of field; because wet collodion plates were used where the emulsion was sensitive to blue and ultraviolet light (which ETW called Actinic rays) he experienced difficulty in determining the correct focus. While he could focus the visible image on the camera glass screen, the actual photographic image would be out of focus because of the high proportion of UV light from the light sources. To overcome this, he calibrated the set-up by exposing plates until he found the optimum focal plane; then he assessed the offset required from the visual focus for each lens and magnification used. ETW termed this a 'turning out' method. Although successful it required considerable dedication and persistence to achieve satisfactory results.

He also experimented with various sources of illumination, including oil, oxy-calcium and magnesium. Using oil, he obtained good results for small enlargements, but the low light output meant exposures of up to 40 minutes and the need for the wet collodion plates to be kept moist using a small vessel of warm water inserted into the camera. Oxy-calcium light produced effective results, but the equipment proved costly, and producing the required oxygen was laborious. ETW's preference was to use magnesium, its only drawback being its lack of 'steadiness': 'if some means could be devised for burning the metal uniformly and at a fixed point', he said, 'nothing would be left to desire.'

ETW also stressed the importance of general care and cleanliness. He advised practitioners to tread lightly, to avoid the slightest vibrations which would disrupt the focus. He stressed the need to avoid the risk of any dust rising and spoiling the end-products. While his design eradicated many of the problems associated with sunlight, other problems arose through the difficulty of having insufficient light and the means to concentrate it. For this method, therefore, it was critical that the ignited strip of magnesium, approximately ¼ inch in length, was placed opposite the pinhole stop (P - see diagram 1) to enable a clear disc of light to be spread evenly over the focusing screen. Another problem arose in determining the required camera lengths for differing degrees of enlargement. This was solved by using a stage micrometer lit by an oil-lamp, rather than the magnesium wire.

In essence, the method may be simplified in the following diagram:

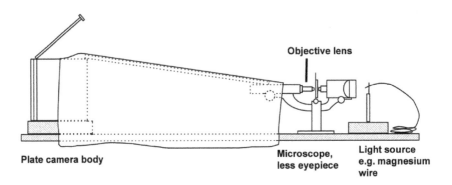

Diagram 2 – A simplified version of the method (courtesy of John White)

Appendix 3 – Statistics showing Cases and Deaths for the Main Diseases Treated at Delancey Hospital

Source: Cheltenham Borough Medical Officer of Health Annual Reports
Note: Statistics of numbers of cases prior to 1890 is inaccurate. More accurate data was only possible following implementation of the Infectious Disease (Notification) Act 1889).

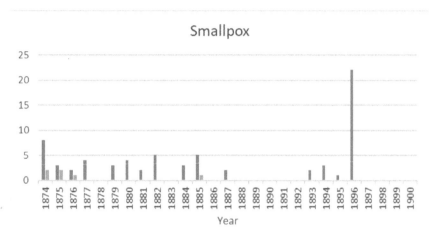

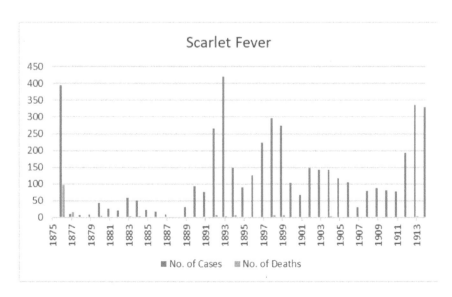

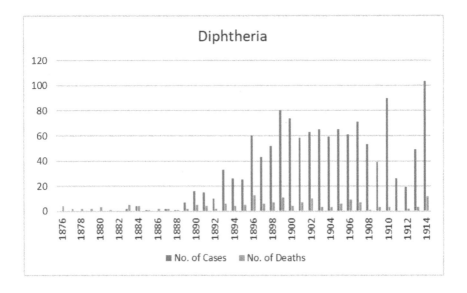

Select Bibliography

This biography has been written using a wide range of primary and secondary sources. Where relevant these have been referenced in the notes for each chapter. Below is a select list of some of the most significant sources that may assist further reading and research.

Primary

a. Archival and unpublished material

Cheltenham Family Welfare Association (formerly the Cheltenham Charities Organisation Society); Cheltenham District Nursing Association. Gloucestershire Archives (Ref. D2465).

Collector Information. Pitt Rivers Museum, University of Oxford.

Delancey Fever Hospital. Gloucestershire Archives (Ref. D3) [includes Trustees' Meeting minutes, 1871-1888, 1896-1948, Management Committee minutes, 1874-1888, 1896-1915, Finance sub-committee minutes 1931-1944, (Ref. D3/1), copy out-correspondence, 1910-1917, (D3/2), bound reports, 1894-1903, unbound reports, 1904-1914, 1916-1935, (Ref. D3/3)].

Double silver chalice inscribed 'General Lord Napier of Magdala RE. to Col R. Woodthorpe RE. to Edward T. Wilson M.B. Oxon. FRCP'. Cheltenham Borough Council and the Cheltenham Trust/The Wilson Family Collection (Ref. 1995.550.229).

Edward Thomas Wilson collection, 1910-1914. The Thomas H. Manning Polar Archives, Scott Polar Research Institute, University of Cambridge (Ref. GB 15 Edward Thomas Wilson).

Minutes books and photographs, Friends in Council Archives.

Recording of an interview between Dr David Wilson and Peter Rendall, together with his sister Betty, at Chippings, 155 The Hill, Burford on 21 September 1996. Cheltenham Borough Council and the Cheltenham Trust/The Wilson Family Collection. (No Ref.).

Student Records, vol. 5 (1855). St George's Hospital, University of London (Ref. SGHMS/4/1/7).

The Great War (1914-1918) letters of E. Bernard Wilson (1868-1950) (Lt. Col. DSO) written home to his family in Cheltenham. Cheltenham Borough Council and the Cheltenham Trust/The Wilson Family Collection. (Ref. 1995.550.77).

Transactions of Cheltenham College Boat Club, 1860. Cheltenham College Archives (Ref. C315/CS).

Wilson, E.T., A single volume of hand-written poems, 1909-1916. Cheltenham Borough Council and the Cheltenham Trust/The Wilson Family Collection (Ref. 1995.550.176).

Wilson, E.T., *Edward Adrian Wilson (1872-1912): a memoir by his father.* Cheltenham Borough Council and the Cheltenham Trust/The Wilson Family Collection (Ref. 1995.550.36).

Wilson, E.T., Extracts of letters, on a single sheet of paper, copied by Edward Thomas Wilson (1832-1918) from Edward Wilson of the Antarctic (1872-1912) to his parents, Cheltenham Borough Council and the Cheltenham Trust/The Wilson Family Collection (Ref. 1995.550.104a).

Wilson, E.T., Letter [to Hunterian Museum], 6 October 1883, Royal College of Surgeons (Ref. RCS-MUS/5/2/4).

Wilson, E.T., *Life of Ted* [early manuscript version]. Cheltenham Borough Council and the Cheltenham Trust/The Wilson Family Collection (Ref. 2010.23).

Wilson, E.T., *My Life. Volume I: 1832-1888. Volume II: 1889-1916.* Illustrated, hand-written. Two black leather volumes with gold lettering. Cheltenham Borough Council and the Cheltenham Trust/The Wilson Family Collection (Ref. 1995.550.35 A & B). [Earlier draft volumes are also available].

Wilson, E.T., 'Record of Family Faculties' [A record of family members and characteristics drafted by Dr E.T.Wilson of Cheltenham (1832-1918) as part of early research into genetic inheritance by Francis Galton FRS]. Cheltenham Borough Council and the Cheltenham Trust/The Wilson Family Collection (Ref. 1995.550.61).

Wilson family of Cheltenham, Gloucestershire Archives (Ref. D10725), 1860s-20th century. [Includes newscuttings books compiled by Dr E.T. Wilson, late 19th century, with index; albums of photographs by E.T. Wilson, 1860s-c.1903; childhood sketchbook of E.A. Wilson, 1870s-1890s; scrapbooks of newscuttings concerning Antarctic expedition, telegrams and letters of condolence sent to Wilson family after E.A. Wilson's death in the Antarctic, 1912; volume of photographs and folder of sketches of Antarctic expedition 1901-1904; pamphlets concerning E.A. Wilson and the Antarctic expedition, 20th century;

'The Alpine Journal' including in memoriam piece on E.A. Wilson, 1913, with newscuttings and letters to Ida Wilson concerning memorial to E.A. Wilson and possible bequest of one of his drawings by her to the Alpine Club, 1957-1958].

b. Publications

Wilson, E.T., 'A national registration of sickness', *British and Foreign Medico-chirurgical Review*, vol. 47 (January-April 1871), pp.396-413.

Wilson, E.T., 'Address by President: Birdnesting', Cheltenham Natural Science Society, 1896.

Wilson, E.T., 'Antarctica', Cheltenham Natural Science Society, 1902.

Wilson, E.T., 'Are small-pox hospitals necessarily (per se) a source of danger to the surrounding population?' [reprinted from the *Transactions of the Society of Medical Officers of Health*], 1885.

Wilson, E.T., 'Death certificates and the registration of disease', *British and Foreign Medico-chirurgical Review*, vol. 44 (July-October 1869), pp.294-315.

Wilson, E.T., *Disinfectants and how to use them*, (H.K. Lewis, [1871]).

Wilson, E.T., 'Distribution of mammalia', Cheltenham Natural Science Society, 1903.

Wilson, E.T., 'Hereditary aptitudes', Cheltenham Natural Science Society, 1891.

Wilson, E.T., 'How to photograph microscopic objects', *The Popular Science Review*, vol. 6 (1867), pp.54-65.

Wilson, E.T., 'Isolation as a means of arresting epidemic disease', *Practitioner* (February 1879), pp.139-160.

Wilson, E.T., 'Man and the extinction of species', Cheltenham Natural Science Society, 1894.

Wilson, E.T., 'Man under evolution', Cheltenham Natural Science Society, 1898.

Wilson, E.T., 'Our flora and fauna: when and whence did they come?', Cheltenham Natural Science Society, 1911.

Wilson, E.T., 'Our inheritance', Cheltenham Natural Science Society, 1910.

Wilson, E.T., 'Photomicrography', *British and Foreign Medico-Chirurgical Review*, vol. 34 (July-October 1864), pp.1-29.

Wilson, E.T., 'Public health', *The Food Journal*, 5 February 1870, pp.31-38 [note: related articles appear in later issues during 1870-72].

Wilson, E.T., 'Public hygiene, and its expositors', *British and Foreign Medico-chirurgical Review*, vol. 53 (January-April 1874), pp.346-65.

Wilson, E.T., 'Questions connected with vaccination' (St George's Hospital Reports), vol. 7 (1872-4), pp.1-15.

Wilson, E.T., 'Sanitary statistics of Cheltenham' in *Report of the Thirty-Fourth Meeting of the British Association for the Advancement of Science held at Bath in September 1864*, (John Murray, 1865), pp.180-183.

Wilson, E.T., 'Sanitary statistics of Cheltenham for the years 1865-71 inclusive', *The British Medical Journal*, 7 September 1872, pp. 268–271.

Wilson, E.T., 'The flints of the Cotteswolds and their uses', Cheltenham Natural Science Society, 1912.

Wilson, E.T., 'The human hand with special reference to finger prints', Cheltenham Natural Science Society, 1907.

Wilson, E.T., 'The limitations of man and how he deals with them', Cheltenham Natural Science Society, 1905.

Wilson, E.T., 'The Long-Barrow Men of the Cotswolds', Cheltenham Natural Science Society, 1913.

Wilson, E.T., 'The mind's eye', Cheltenham Natural Science Society, 1884.

Wilson, E.T., 'The plague of 1871 in Buenos Ayres', *The Food Journal*, vol.3 (1 February 1872), pp.19-22.

Wilson, E.T., 'The President's Address read 15 October 1891', Cheltenham Natural Science Society, 1891.

Wilson, E.T., 'Thoughts on the cosmos', Cheltenham Natural Science Society, 1904.

Wilson, E.T., 'Whales', Cheltenham Natural Science Society, 1901.

Wilson, E.T. and Sawyer, J. (Eds.), *A Guide to Cheltenham* (British Medical Association. Cheltenham Meeting, 1901), (Norman, Sawyer and Co., 1901).

Secondary

Beale, L.S., *How to work with the microscope* (Harrison 1868), 4th ed., pp.247-249.

Cardew, G. A., *Echoes and reminiscences of medical practitioners in Cheltenham of the nineteenth century*, (Ed J Burrow & Co Ltd, 1930).

Committee of the Entomological Society of Philadelphia, *A Memoir of Thomas Bellerby Wilson*, (The Entomological Society of Philadelphia, 1865).

Dudgeon, J.A., 'Development of smallpox vaccine in England in the eighteenth and nineteenth centuries', *British Medical Journal* (25 May 1963), pp.1367-1372.

Elder, D. 'Dr Edward T. Wilson', in Prowse, S. (ed.), *Capturing the moment: 150 years of photography in Cheltenham*, (Cheltenham Camera Club, 2015), pp.14-21.

Elder, D., 'Edward T. Wilson (1832-1918) co-founder of Cheltenham Photographic Society, *Cheltenham Local History Society Journal*, vol. 24 (2008), pp.3-9.

Elder, D. '"He went about doing good": the life of Dr. Edward Thomas Wilson (1832-1918)', *Cheltenham Local History Society Journal*, vol. 22 (2006), pp.13-21.

MacInnes, K., *Woman with the iceberg eyes: Oriana F. Wilson*, (The History Press, 2019).

Miller, E. 'Dr Wilson and his friends', *Cheltenham Local History Society Journal*, vol. 35 (2019), pp.12-15.

O'Connor, D. and Harvey, I. *Troubled waters: the great Cheltenham water controversy*, (David A. O'Connor, 2007).

Savours, A. (ed.), *Edward Wilson: Diary of the Discovery expedition to the Antarctic regions 1901-1904*, (Blandford Press, 1966).

Seaver, G., *Edward Wilson of the Antarctic: naturalist and friend*, (John Murray, 1933).

Snook, M. *Wolseley, Wilson and the failure of the Khartoum Campaign: an exercise in scapegoating and abrogation of command responsibility?* PhD thesis, (Cranfield University, 2004).

Watson, C.M. *The life of Major-General Sir Charles Wilson*, (John Murray, 1909).

Whishaw, J., *A history of the Whishaw family*, (Methuen, 1935).

Wildman, S., *Local nursing associations in an age of nursing reform, 1860-1900*. PhD thesis, (University of Birmingham, 2012).

William Osler, Bibliotheca Osleriana: a catalogue of books illustrating the history of medicine and science, (McGill-Queen's University Press, 1969), p.687. [Index entry for ETW is 7633].

Wilson, D.M. and Elder, D.B., *Cheltenham in Antarctica: the life of Edward Wilson*, (Reardon Publishing, 2000).

Wilson, E. *Diary of the Terra Nova expedition to the Antarctic 1910-1912*, (Blandford Press, 1972).

Index

References which include illustrations are given in bold.

Lightning Source UK Ltd.
Milton Keynes UK
UKHW020648261121
394627UK00002B/8